SAME PATH,
Different Shoes

V.J. Norton

Grosvenor House
Publishing Limited

The right of V.J. Norton to be identified as the author of this
work has been asserted in accordance with Section 78
of the Copyright, Designs and Patents Act 1988

The book cover picture is copyright to http://www.123rf.com/profile_hibrida

This book is published by
Grosvenor House Publishing Ltd
Link House
140 The Broadway, Tolworth, Surrey, KT6 7HT.
www.grosvenorhousepublishing.co.uk

A CIP record for this book
is available from the British Library

ISBN 978-1-78623-824-5

Acknowledgments

A special dedication to the late Eileen Lockett OBE who worked tirelessly for Cancer Research.

All the Metropolitan Police Officers in Waltham Forest, the dedicated members of staff at Flint House Police Rehabilitation Centre and for those who have suffered, been diagnosed or have cared for those suffering from cancer, let my story be an inspiration to you, your friends and your family.

As contentious as this book may be, it is based on my true-life experience, as I too battled against breast cancer.

A special thank you to my rock David, Samantha, Alexander, Mum, Shirley and of course my diamond sister-in-law Kate Norton, for cheering me on every step of the way (and tactfully not asking me how it was going too often).

Thank you to my friends and family; we have grown closer and tighter together with real love. The bubble we have formed has shielded us from the negativities of the outside world.

A note from Verna

I never set out to write a book about cancer. The truth is, I've never really seen myself as a writer.

When I told my son and daughter that I was writing a book, they both said, "Wow Mum, that's great. What are you going to say?"

My stories have turned me on enough to get me to dedicate seven months of my time. Unique for me as a writer and hopefully unique to you, as a reader.

Please allow me to share my empowering journey with you.

Cancer. The disease. The big C. That thing. Cancer, the forbidden word.

Cancer, the killer that comes upon you like a thief in the night.

No rhyme or reason, it chooses randomly and will attempt to take over unless you get equipped to fight this deadly disease.

In truth, my reason for writing this book is to share my fight with you. I was betrayed into thinking that I was healthy. No lump, no symptoms could indicate that breast cancer was developing and multiplying inside of me. It was only through requesting a routine mammogram that I shockingly discovered that I had early stage breast cancer.

This book is based on my true story. The names have been changed to protect the identity of the characters that appear in this book.

I have compressed certain time periods and altered the identity and background of certain individuals so that they would not be recognisable.

Prologue

"Ashes to ashes, dust to dust," proclaimed the man with the wavy dark hair and dark cloak, as he stood draped over me like a hawk.

I could hear the sounds of weeping in the background.

He raised his hands to his shoulders, gently levering as he sprinkled gravel over my soul.

The grit of the pattering soil was quickly drowning me. It felt as though I was sinking in quicksand. My body lay heavy and helpless as I tried to call out.

My vision was gradually fading.

My voice was silent despite desperately shouting and screaming out, "Please, help. Help me." I was being covered in fresh soil, which was weighing me down. The weight of the earth became heavier and heavier.

My time on earth was moving more and more into the distance.

I could still hear the voices and echoes of the mourners. I heard the pain and the sorrow of their grieving.

"Stop. Please stop. Stop." I pleaded.

Ping!

Startled, I asked myself what was going on. I started shivering as I grasped the duvet covers. My hair stuck together like mounded lard and I reached up and touched my neck, which was dripping with sweat.

I rubbed the sleep from my eyes as I tried desperately to focus, flickering my eyelids. There was no movement in the room.

The darkness was filled with silence.

I reached over to my left side to feel for my mobile phone. I fumbled over using my fingertips and felt a smooth sharp cold object. Ouch! That wasn't it. I continued moving my fingertips cautiously. I felt the flat surface and picked it up by the smooth edge and pressed the groove. The glare was so bright, I flipped the phone to its back and blocked it until my eyes adjusted. 03.27 am.

Gosh is that all…

I looked around; it was still dark.

I looked up to the ceiling and felt a great sense of euphoria.

"Lord," I cried out, "Did you call me?"

I waited for a few seconds. What was I saying, I thought.

Uncontrollably the words come out again, "Lord, did you call me?" My mouth was dribbling. I rubbed my eyes with both hands to see if there was anyone there.

I heard a distorted, unrecognisable deep male voice whisper, "Child, continue to live your life. I am not ready for you yet."

"Hey you! I need a face to face," I shouted. "Come again!" I was feeling confident as I braced myself for a reaction.

Growing up

My story wouldn't be complete without a little insight into my world growing up. I was born in Tottenham, North London and grew up in the Windrush era of the 1960-70s. Raised within a multi-occupancy household with my mother, Ivy Pearl Petgrave, the late Noel Petgrave and my sister Shirley, I remember my parents living in a one bedroomed room. It was like a studio flat, situated on the top floor within a large eight bedroomed house in The Avenue, Tottenham.

My father worked as a barber – yes, typical of the character in the TV sitcom *Desmond's* – he would entertain his customers with his huge personality, share his stories and a joke or two. Being in Dad's shop was his show, his arena. The customers would either wait hours for a haircut or just pop in for the entertainment. During the show, Dad would often pop out leaving his clients still strapped in the chair whilst he placed a bet or two at his local bookies.

Mum worked part time in the bingo hall in Bruce Grove and they both worked tirelessly to feed and clothe us and pay the rent. I often remember having to keep quiet at certain knocks on the door, not sure if it was the insurance man or rent man, but I quickly learned the rules; I would look to my mother's eyes for direction. "Shoo shoosh," she would say as she held her forefinger up to her lips and stared at me intensely. I got the message, no questions were asked.

There was a huge sense of relief when the footsteps of big boots would fade away. "Phew," a sigh of relief as we carried on our chores until next Thursday.

1

I would often be privy to conversations about the racism often experienced and spoken about by my parents and their friends. It was a normal expectation, a sort of way of life as they struggled to be accepted and integrate in their chosen new life in Britain. Great Britain.

It was usual for big prams to be left outside shops as mothers would congregate for discussions and gossip. There was no such awareness of child abduction or at least it was rare. Prams were big and grand therefore had to be left outside in the front gardens of premises. There were no fold up or downs and were often used as transportation for other children, shopping and coal.

Iron stoves would be a common feature on the balconies for cooking. You would often feed the meter a shilling at a time, but by the time you came to cook your own meals for yourself and your family you often found you had to refill the meter with another shilling as the previous occupant would make full use of your credit.

A shilling was a lot of money in those days, equivalent to a shopping basket for a bag of rice, a tub of Bovril and a packet of cornmeal for porridge. My mother recalls the milkman would deliver the red and gold top milk and I would choose the red top as I liked the colour so much and bring it upstairs for her.

I got a great sense of the tension felt and a flavour of the frustrations felt by the community. It seems that you would have to curb your tongue. Your tolerance levels were at a peak as you tried to make a success of your life in England and yearn to be accepted within this society. It was a cheek by jowl existence.

You were really grateful to have a roof over your head. You would wash your clothes by hand and laundry in the bath was common place. You would then place your clothes inside your room on your clothes rail. Mum said it was not nice, but it was a start to a better life. All the tenants were in the same position as you, therefore you quickly adapted to a queuing method of living, adjusting quickly in desperation to conform to a new and better life.

In those days white folks would not rent any houses or rooms to black people full stop. There were notices on the front doors or windows. 'No Blacks. No Irish. No Dogs.'

I suppose, as folk got more used to immigration they became more accepting and tolerant. As time went by the notices would slowly disappear from the doors and windows, but when you knocked on the door the occupants looked at you sympathetically and would politely say, 'Sorry darling, no vacancies.'

Mum says that the response would be almost one of empathy. A well-rehearsed short announcement. No hard feelings, love!

No one was prepared to bend the rules overtly, but I do wonder, could this have been the start of the sudden surge of mixed race babies coming to the fore...

As you travelled from door to door, a sense of patriotism was felt. You were welcomed by your own ethnic background. They would be more obliging, after all they had made it in England and became the landlords. A sense of 'help me out, bruv' was felt.

In those days, you did not have the luxury of radiators, you had just paraffin heaters in your room, you would purchase the oil from the local garage and struggle to get it home. Sometimes the huge canister would take the place of the babies in the prams, there were no health and safety rules then.

As a child I recall listening and learning life skills quickly at an early age.

To be told once was enough, otherwise there were life threatening consequences. You were fascinated by the flaming lights of the fire in your family packed room often filled with the aroma of poisonous fumes of paraffin gases. You touched, you would burn; it was a simple as that.

I remember being entertained by watching the flicker of the red and orange flames, coated with blue. I would place both hands out for warmth. I remember standing up with my back against the fire, as I turned around I was careful not to touch the fire, the warm feeling on my back and the back of my legs was bliss.

The heat of the caged door would indicate if I was too near or not. If you touched it by either curiosity or any accident that was it, mate, you got burnt. Tough luck. Simply don't do it again!

The saying, 'If you can't hear, you must feel,' prevailed.

Later on in my youth I recall sitcoms such as *Love Thy Neighbour*, *Mind Your Language* and *Rising Damp*. I suppose it was accepted as funny and innovative, perhaps funny enough to break down the barriers within the different races; as folk mingled, tolerance was filtered through comedy.

The barriers slowly broke down over the decades and attitudes changed for the better.

I recall introducing my first friend from school to my mother and father.

Mum, Dad, this is Jane.

They delightfully looked her up and down; they approved. She was my next door neighbour, She had porcelain white skin, blonde stringy hair like hay and blue eyes that resembled sapphires. We believed that this integration was the beginning of being united.

Growing up, we didn't see colour or race, However, I do recall once holding hands as we skipped to the playground. Our clasps would tighten as we turned our hands around and compared the contrast. No words were spoken, there was no need. As far as we were concerned we were friends and we were going to have lots of fun.

I remember holding hands as we sought adventures, playing hopscotch and run outs, to name a few. We enjoyed our friendship, and would look forward to seeing each other everyday.

I remember frowning at the thought of being called indoors by either of our parents right in the middle of a game, or being told that we had to go and visit relatives. Drat! I remember feeling really cheated and feeling that life was so unfair. I don't think my parents understood how important friendship was when you are young and carefree or perhaps they had simply forgotten.

We were very privileged to live within a household of other West Indian occupants. They too were from the West Indies; these Windrush recruits sought hope and a better life. They were full of beans and enthusiasm, this was their dream, this was our future.

The man who was that passenger at the back of the bus is now driving the bus. That woman who was taking her children for their inoculations was now administering them as a nurse. Their dreams came true.

Mum and Dads friends were mainly of Irish and Cypriot descent. Dad often spoke so highly of his friends Paddy and Deidra. Mum often spoke of her late friend Alexandra.

Paddy was a thick set Irish builder with red hair and a black heavy donkey jacket and denim jeans. I don't recall him wearing anything other than this style. He would often reek of alcohol and share jokes and work experiences with Dad as they filled the room with roars of laughter.

Deidra was a typical Irish nurse, gentle and caring. She had a secret lover from the West Indies and became pregnant with his child, whom she brought up as a single parent. He was already married and she was his bit on the side.

She embraced the West Indian culture, and had a twang in her accent that really resembled a West Indian accent – a mixture of accents that somehow mingled together into a tranquil whole, hilarious!

She would shop for curry goat with my mother and they would cook rice and peas and chicken with all the spices, which perfected any authentic West Indian cooking. Her daughter, Miranda was a precious jewel to her and her partner, this secret would be most unwelcome by her Irish folks back home. Sadly Miranda's existence was hidden, therefore she had no cousins or grandparents or other relatives in her life.

This relationship had to be kept secret to prevent Deidra being disowned by her family and also prevent her elderly parents and relatives from suffering a serious illness through the shock of knowing that their daughter had deceived them in their eyes and had engaged in an interracial relationship and worse of all produced a mixed-race child; this was equally as serious as committing a murder.

Alexandra resided in England for some twenty years. Again, I suppose for a better life. She and her husband emigrated from Cyprus and raised their family alongside ours, we were all immigrants together. Alexandra always wore black clothing; she had dark curly hair, clear olive skin and a beard. Yes, she would kiss me and it was all spiky, I dreaded it.

You would think that Alexandra came to England under duress. She refused to learn the English language. Surprisingly, we somehow managed to communicate with her generosity of kindness, delicious Greek food and damn good company.

If she felt like it, she would make an effort with her children interpreting when she was lost for the correct words and terminology. This would often make me smirk and I would find myself holding my stomach in my ultimate efforts to disguise my belly laughs.

In frustration, she would shout, 'Fucking bastards!' After all, she was rebel without a cause from Cyprus. I suppose she didn't want to let go of her culture or her identity.

The integration amongst the Blacks, Irish, Asian and any person really not considered to be English was hard; we were all competing to be the accepted race.

Friday nights were party night in our house. The fun and great expectations of the Friday night parties made the weekends. The old reggae artists such as Toots and the Maytals, Jimmy Cliff and Pat Kelly's *How Long Will It Take?* and *Talk About Love* would be blaring out through the Formica homemade speakers patched up with plywood and vinyl. I would secretly pretend to be asleep when I heard Mum's footsteps, as she sneaked upstairs to check on me and my sister. I would place the pink cellular blanket over my face with one eye peeping out.

I would watch her with excitement as she carefully tiptoed on her stiletto heels in an effort not to wake us, the scent of Sweet Aurora perfume filled the room. I would watch in admiration as she pulled the light switch on the dressing table to check her makeup and touched up her lippy and face powder. I would watch her secretly as I tried so hard not to giggle. She would make weird faces and expressions in the mirror, her trout pout was definitely original. When finished she had gained the satisfaction and confidence to return downstairs to join the other partygoers. The stairs would creak as she crept downstairs one by one in this three-storey Victorian detached house.

Full of excitement and a sense of escapism she would tootle back downstairs the floor boards creaked with her every step and this faded as she got nearer. I would hear a rush of noise filled with laughter and delight and the door would then be closed shut.

This was my go ahead to throw the blanket to the side, jump out of bed and creep downstairs.

I would carefully open the door ajar and observe my mum and dad, the great hosts. They both danced to perfection as though they were competitors in a *Strictly Come Dancing* tournament. Cheers of encouragement from the spectators were reassuringly loud with strong accents. The culture from back home was filled with booze, fags and dancing.

I witnessed some serious skilled body moves, twisting and jiving coupled with very talented dancing. *Strictly Come Dancing* would definitely have been met with some serious competition.

Mum and Dad would show off their dancing skills and my Uncle Doc, Dalton and Auntie Anne would then compete to beat them by bettering their skills. The room was filled with tobacco smoke, jeers and laughter. Pet nicknames were used to refer to each other, the names were transferred from back home, Dad's was Bobsy the Beaver. When he danced they would cheer and shout, 'Hallo! Gwan Beaver!'

His confidence grew more and more as he raised his head to the ceiling with pride, his neck would extend as he added in a twist to his hips and that extra step or two in his steps as a bonus.

After the heat of this spectacular show he would reach to his back pocket for his handkerchief to wipe his brow, before replacing it in his back pocket again for another performance. I would watch with pride and admiration.

The name Beaver derived from when he was a young buddying barber in Portland, Jamaica. When he arrived to take up his transferable skills in England, Bobsy the barber had made it. I am told that he inherited the name because of his bandy bowed legs and the fact that he was an amazing swimmer.

My mother Ivy was a country bumpkin from Clarendon, Jamaica – a very shy and loyal mother who doted on me and my sister.

I smile fondly at the memories of yesterday's ska and reggae, Desmond Dekker *Ah It Mek* and Jimmy Cliff *The Harder They Come* blaring from the record player, for them a reminder of home. The Jamaican rum and coke and a full pot of curry goat and rice 'n peas to share; everything was 'Ire'.

It was usual to dance with contentment, even without the sound of any music playing; dancing was the freeing and liberating of one soul with a sense of pride.

In the mornings I would often volunteer to assist my mum in clearing up from the night before.

I'd carefully watch Mum turn her head to any distraction and use this opportunity to quickly gulp the remains of last night's delights, vodka and orange cordial, rum and coke and brandy and lemonade. Do you think this could have been my introduction to alcohol? I ask, tongue in cheek!

In the 70s we fortunately qualified for a brand new council flat. No more cold taps, stove ovens and going to the toilet in the back garden's cold and dark outdoor toilet.

We lived on the sixth floor in White Hart Lane directly overlooking the Spurs ground. In those days you could look out of your balcony and watch the football match. We were rich, we had everything you could dream of.

Health and happiness, our wooden spoon was the equivalent of your silver spoon. Tottenham Comprehensive School was the local school; there was no such thing as catchment areas, you just simply went to the nearest school.

We would attend the local outfitters who would issue the blazer, school badge, shirt, tie and all the other outfits. September was always an exciting time to return to school after the break of the summer holidays.

I considered myself as an average student, with a very artistic streak, not a popular student but, under the radar I would say. Miraculously, somehow I still managed to bring myself to the attention of the school bullies, perhaps through my choice of dress, skinny stature, cockney accent or I suppose my eccentric personality. I dared to be different and still do.

I became more confident with my image, I began smoking cigarettes at the age of 13, this was so cool, I would take puffs behind the bike sheds at school and even in the school toilets before being flushed out by the head of year, Ms Hunt, Sergeant Major!!

I would shave the sides of my hair and dyed my hair red in my effort to make a personal statement. I would loosen my school tie, fold my skirt waistband band twice over my waist in my poor efforts to create a miniskirt effect and to complete the style I placed two of dad's socks in my bra, 32AA. I became funky and stylish in my own right.

I drew the friends that were left over for me, the ones that were considered to be the overspill of the goody two shoe gang and the ones not quite bad or horrid enough to be part of the school bullies.

Today I still have many meaningful and fond relationships with my old school friends who will always hold a special place in my heart. Here I go spilling my emotions again...

Upon reaching the age of seventeen years, my parents divorced. I could not understand why my father would leave my beautiful mother for another. I wonder now if it was a midlife crisis.

When he did return home, it would be for a change of clothing or to quickly grab some of his personal belongings. I remember a short encounter having waited for him to return home to see us, sometimes two or three days later. He was always well groomed and reeked of aftershave. I remember thinking that he was having so much more fun than us. He was out and about in his car with his friends, while we were stuck at home living by orders and rules.

Mum turned to religion, it was never going to be the same. It got better as she prayed for us, her daughters everyday.

My sister suffered a short illness and was consequently left profoundly deaf. I felt that I had taken Dad's place indirectly; I would become the stronger one of the two and would often be relied upon to fill in forms and facilitate communications on behalf of my mother and sister. I followed instructions from my mother to perfection, well there was no other choice. I became the more dominant member of my family, when I left school I knew exactly where I wanted to go and who I wanted to be.

I always worked upon leaving school at 15 years of age. That's one of the privileges of having an August birthday, you are forever young I am told.

Jobs ranged from the sweet factories in Broad Lane, Tottenham, to a bakery assistant in my local Tesco's in Edmonton Green.

I also enjoyed working in a chocolate factory, Jameson in Northumberland Park after school; all the locals worked there, a real local community environment. I would finish school and clock in taking over from my mum's shift; she would then go home to prepare dinner for the evening.

I have extremely fond memories working in Manzes Pie and Mash shop in Islington, my friend Candice owned it with her husband Colin.

It was such a novelty at the time, the only black female to work in a traditional pie and mash shop serving up jellied eels. I quickly learned how to make pies and liquor and there was definitely a place for my cockney accent and this became complete to perfection, an accent I have not managed to shake off very well.

In my first proper job I worked as a girl Friday for a toy company called D Dekkers, a foundation for my customers service status before progressing as a back office dealing clerk for Barclays Bank in Gracechurch Street, London. It was so cool being a city girl in the booming 1980s.

I worked tirelessly to complete the daily deadlines of huge CHAPs payments for large purchases. The pressures grew with the demands of the job and culture, my competitive nature peaked as I became more confident and influential. I loved everything about the buzz of working in the City of London. I felt a sense of achievement and I would often quietly reaffirm, 'The girl from Nam, has done well'.

I have fond memories of meetings over Leadenhall market for lunches after work, drinking champagne, discovering the delights of Dom Perignon champagne, regular meeting in wine bars and through over-intoxication flaking out in local hotel rooms, as I was often too worse for wear to travel back home.

My bank balance would often take a hammering as I added to my wide variety of cassette tape collections – George Michael, Madonna and Whitney Houston were worth the struggle. I would often cling to the last pennies of my overdraft to get me through to pay day.

I was in a new circle, I liked it and it was full of inspiration. I practiced and practiced to perfection my speech to speak more refined. I couldn't afford elocution lessons so I just practiced "Yah, darling. Yah, Yah, Yah!" It became natural, becoming more plum and refined like my colleagues, who either came from Essex or the other side of South London, south somewhere... I suppose in the suburbs.

I discovered my natural ability to change and adapt to suit my audiences and would often practice and practice to perfection. I was able to switch automatically from my work colleagues' 'toodle pips' to my sister's 'Raaaahh' – that's what you call real adaptable talent!

"Essex, where the hell is that?" I asked, mainly intrigued and puzzled, I could feel my forehead creasing to portray the validity and seriousness of the question being asked.

Penny, my colleague explained that she actually came from a place called Canvey Island, Where the fuck was that? I had visions of an island on its own in the middle of nowhere full of posh white people surrounded by a river and you would have to travel by boat to get there.

I bought my first flat and moved from Tottenham to a flat in Walthamstow and then progressed to a two-up two-down house.

I quickly met my husband and after a short romance married; two children later, I became a mother and wife with real responsibilities.

My youth was quickly shortened; I had to grow up now. I became a responsible adult prematurely cut in my prime; this I blame for my immature nature.

I took pride flouncing the sparkling rock on my wedding finger. It was goodbye to those of you who took my heart and stored it in your sweets jar, it was now too late.

We moved to Chigwell, my parents were very proud and I would often hear my dad boasting to his clients in his shop when he thought I was out of earshot. I would hear him say, "She has done well, she is not living around here, you know. She has bought a house in the country." There would often be three men waiting in a line as customers, together they would nod in agreement, as though acknowledging the words of a preacher at Sunday morning church. They must have heard the same line over and over again.

Mum would do the same to her church sisters and brothers, always praising how well we had done. The look of affirmation, approval and respect felt like receiving a radar of positive vibes of beaming energy.

My husband doted on us, his dream family. My daughter Samantha Holly was born on Christmas Day, 13months later my son Alexander David was born January new year of 1992.

After a big career change decision, I decided to join the Police Service. After seeing the children through their teenage years, I pursued my career choice and was very proud and honoured to belong and I wore the uniform with great pride.

I trained at Hendon Police School and my probation can only be described as like adult boarding school. I was later posted to Waltham Forest as a sworn Police Constable, a very touching proud moment for me and my family.

This proved to be one of the best decisions I have made in my life. I swear to you, I have worked amongst the most dedicated caring professionals you could ever imagine. Some of you can verify this, because I have taken you out on patrol with me. You too have witnessed the professionalism and experienced the ooze of enthusiasm.

Father passed away peacefully in 2004; I remain full of gratitude and thanks that his life was spared timely.

We were blessed that he had a relationship with his grandchildren and saw me grow older. The children referred to him as Granddad Cut/Cut, the well-known barber within his community. They looked up to their granddad.

He was spared the opportunity to witness his daughter patrol the streets of Waltham Forest as a fully pledged sworn-in uniformed Police Officer before quietly falling asleep.

Due to the empathy and kindness of my superiors at that time of sorrow and pain, my colleagues organised the smooth procession of his funeral. It was their duty as colleagues, which they carried out with pride.

On the day of his funeral, the colourful steel band paraded through Forest Road Walthamstow. It was like a royal occasion as the bearers walked step by step with their sticks in tune to the beat of the band and the horses were well behaved with their feather dressings. Typical way to go Dad, hope this did you proud.

What a moment, I bet you never thought you would go out like this Dad, did you?

A toast to you, the greatest love of my life.

After two years as a probationer I graduated to a Detective Constable where I undertook a range of very interesting roles.

I found it only right and natural to build a rapport straight away and adapt to many situations. I was always a fair cop... don't commit the crime if you can't do the time.

Well I am from 'Nam after all! I know how things run. This reaffirmation was an asset and has kept me well grounded.

The M-word

Flint House, Goring

14th December 2015 was the date I was given for my rehabilitation. My blood pressure was playing hide and seek with me, one day it would be 130, next day for no reason it would be 180. I needed time out from work to recharge my batteries.

Bloody hell, why then? It's too late in the year, why couldn't they have given me a summer date, I thought as I prepared myself for two weeks of rehab.

As I packed I was a bit apprehensive about leaving home, but I was so exhausted and was feeling rather peaky, partly due to my high blood pressure and excessive weight that had crept up around my fat belly over the years. I suppose it was the calm before the storm of Christmas 2015.

Before I zipped closed my suitcase, I found a small bottle of brandy looking at me.

17th December 2015, part of the rehabilitation process incorporated a routine medical health check up.

I arrived for my appointment and was greeted by Nurse Christine Lacey. She welcomed me into her sterile consultation room where I was immediately put at ease. She was warm and easy to speak to, she had a very soft gently nature, it's almost as though she was an angel sent to watch over me.

We spoke about my family and children; she then gently pulled my arm towards her and checked my blood pressure, then my BMI and cholesterol. She directed me to the weighing scales. On route, I declared, "I know, I know, I have a fat belly and I need cut down on wine and stop smoking, I will lose weight and be healthier." But my mind shied away from that, flinching at the idea.

"Yes, yes I will definitely try."

She smiled and waited for me to finish my sentence. She then replied, "Verna I am not here to lecture you, you are already aware of some of the detriments these things can have on your health."

"Yep, that's fine," I said as I nodded in acknowledgment to confirm to her that I was taking this on board.

I could cope with this constructive criticism and skilfully diverted the conversation, "Yes I do try to look after myself, I drink plenty of water and keep up to date with my health check appointments, smears etc."

I then noticed that I was rambling on before being interrupted.

"Have you had a mammogram?"

"No," I replied. "What's that?"

"Well it's a service that is offered to check your breasts," she said. "Do you check your breasts?" she asked.

"Yes I do," as I proudly reached to my breast to demonstrate to her, I raised my arms and rubbed my breast under my arms to show my competence.

"Good," she said and produced leaflets and useful guides on breast self-examination techniques.

As I left the consultation room with the leaflets, something was bugging me…

Mammogram… It detects early breast cancer. It kept going over and over in my mind.

I thought of all the people known to me suffering from cancer. I'd be a fool not to pursue this.

A mammogram, I've heard of it but was not sure of the process. No, I thought as I heeded the advice offered. I said to myself, I want one of those.

A mammogram, a mammogram. This kept on cropping up in my mind.

Later on that evening, it was about 8pm. I settled down for the evening in my single room. I got my diary out and in the diary I entered 5th January 2016.

I thought to myself I will get Christmas over and done with and then revisit this date 5th January 2016, I will then make enquires and have a mammogram.

For those of you that know me, you know that I do note everything down in my little blue book; little did I know that this note of entry was the one that was about to save my life.

Gatekeeper

The 5th January 2016.

I called my local GP.

"Doctors Surgery, Mrs Gatekeeper speaking," the voice answered.

"Hello, would you be kind enough to book me a mammogram appointment please."

Mrs Gatekeeper, the doctor's receptionist asked me the following – it was almost as though she was reading from a scroll on the wall, you know the ones, jobsworth...

"Have you found a lump?"

I replied "No."

"Do you feel unwell?"

"No," I replied.

"Well," she said, "why do you want a mammogram?"

"Well, I have just been recommended for one and I want one please."

I could hear Mrs Gatekeeper tap in her computer and after a few seconds she diverted her attention back to me on the telephone.

"Due to an administration error we have not got you on the list, and in any case you have now missed the round up of patients being called up for this service. You will have to wait for the next round to be called up."

There were no signs or symptoms of this silent killer to substantiate my case. This gut feeling overtook me; the more Mrs Gatekeeper was telling me no, the more I was insistent and said yes. I insisted in having it, my gut instincts said yes, yes, yes... I will get this somehow...

"Listen here, I know too many people that have left it too late. One in three of us women will suffer from some form of cancer, who are you to prevent this, my right?" I felt like a terrier gnashing at the feet of someone who had my bone and was waving it in front of me.

"Listen," she replied, almost as though she had been defeated, "there are no appointments in Redbridge," begrudgingly she said, "here is the telephone number for Epping St. Margaret's. Call them and see what they have to offer."

Thank you, Mrs Gatekeeper, you indirectly preserved my life.

After a tiresome presentation of my case on the phone to Epping St Margaret, I secured an appointment. My voice must have sounded intensely desperate, the receptionist Mrs Cando secured a suitable appointment.

I secured a mammogram appointment, which appeared safely in my blue book and I wrote down the date given as 5th January 2016.

On the morning of my appointment, I confidently ticked off the date, mission accomplished.

I arrived and was very nervous and apprehensive, I didn't know what to expect, I mean I had seen programmes on TV and magazine features, but I hadn't really given it much attention before now.

The lady asked me to take off my top and bra, as I did this I went in to auto pilot. I stood in front of this big apparatus with metal cups, I stood there puzzled as the lady explained to me from the other side of the apparatus what was going to happen.

Oh my God what an experience, each breast in turn squashed in to this damn square-shaped metal device, I couldn't believe what was happening, I thought this was some kind of sick joke. As the nurse repeated this process, she acknowledged how uncomfortable it was and continued to assist me in squeezing my breast in turn in what I can only describe as a first taste of a torture chamber.

She must have had this herself or taken on board the feedback from previous patients in order to offer me the kind of empathy and reassurance that she provided. I was so relieved when this was over and done.

Done it. Dun it, dun it. Had the mammogram, that's the end of that, so I thought; little did I expect to be recalled a week later.

The Letter

"Verna, Verna, are you OK? I think you are having a bad dream..."

I smelt that sweet scent of fresh lilies as the duvet was placed snugly over my shoulders and warms lips that sealed the kiss reassured me that I was in safe hands.

Silence filled the room... I knew as soon as I woke up that it was going to be a very special day,

I looked admiringly at my new shoes, the ones that I had bought yesterday. Yes the ones that sent me into my overdraft, I just had to have them. I stared at them from the corner of the room as I imagined myself walking tall in them, this filled me with excitement, the autumn sunlight streamed through the rattan blinds, gliding the bedsheets back I could smell the rain that had fallen in the night, and see the leaves on the plane tree in the garden below, just turning golden brown at the tips.

I closed my eyes again and stretched, listening to the tick and groan of the heating, and the muted roar of traffic, feeling every muscle, revelling in the day to come.

I always start my mornings in the same way. Maybe it's something about the kids being off your hands. You are able to get set in your ways, there are no outside disruptions, no flatmates to hoover up after, no cat coughing up a hairball on the rug. You have an idea of what you left in the cupboard the night before will be in the cupboard when you wake up. You're in control.

I felt alone with the voices in my head, the characters I had created. The silence became so real.

Having a routine is important and to keep a diary is equally important. It gives you something to hang on to, something to differentiate the weekdays from the weekends.

At 6.30am exactly the heating went on, the roar of the boiler always wakes me up.

I looked at my phone – just to check the world had not ended without me and then lay there listening to the pop and creak of the radiator.

I levered myself out of my warm duvet and grabbed my dressing gown.

I walked over to the corner of the room and tried my new shoes on. I looked down and turned the heels sideward before placing my feet firmly on the ground. I looked in the mirror and admired the sparkle of my new shoes.

I flipped them off before running down three flights of stairs. I switch on the coffee maker that is preloaded with coffee and water the night before.

The coffee is usually through by the time I have read my emails and plan for the day.

I reached for my diary, I had a mammogram appointment booked for 10.30am.

I pulled on a t-shirt, some leggings and socks and shoved my feet into my trainers where I'd left them near the door and went out into the world.

Off I went to the gym.

When I got back, I was hot and sweating and loose limbed with tiredness and I stood for a long time under the shower, thinking about my to do list for the day. I wasn't due in work until 14.00.

I needed to do another online shop and I was nearly out of food.

Shit it's 10.15, I need to get to Epping by 10.30am.

I had the mammogram and for the next few days, I put it out of my mind. I busied myself with work and socialising with friends.

A week later a letter from the health trust arrived.

"Verna, a letter has come from the hospital."

I sat frowning at the letter, chewing the side of my gum before opening it.

Oh, I thought as I opened the letter, my stomach dropped as I read the first lines. I read the letter again to make sense of it. When it finally sunk in I gathered that I was being recalled for further tests due to abnormalities detected in my right breast. How the hell did that get there?

Could it be a mistake? Had they plundered their database and fired off letters to anyone they could find.

One in three are detected for having cancer, that meant that my inclusion could hardly be a mistake. Right?

What the fuck, was this normal, I asked myself. I looked at Dave, we did not say anything, there was DOUBT, but we were both too scared to say anymore.

"I'll come with you next week, I've got the time off work."

We both attended the hospital where I underwent further mammograms, the surgeon confirmed that there were abnormalities, again squashed my breasts to a pulp with the cold metal plates. I then had to have a biopsy which was very, very painful, it felt as though a staple gun was being administered four times in a row. This was to identify what the abnormalities were.

Lymph nodes and nuclear tests were given and there was a cold chilling feeling going through my veins and numerous blood test to include testing for the sickle cell gene.

An angiogram, which picked up a dormant hernia was amongst other exhausting gruelling and painful of tests.

At this stage I detached my soul from my body, this was to help me to block out what I was about to undergo. I was just a shell that sacrificed my broken body.

It was as suspected, my nightmare began. Early stage breast cancer in my right breast, there was no mistake and no error.

This beast did not form a lump. It did not make me feel ill or sick. It did not show its ugly face but it was killing me very slowly.

At this stage, this was not wholly confirmed but heavily suspected, sadly I could not see any glimmer of hope.

A nightmare scenario had begun, whether I was ready or not and without any choice I was playing the leading role. It felt as though it was raining all over the world for days.

The feeling of utter pain and helplessness prevailed.

When I was a child I used to play 'it' and run away. Now I was 'it' and there was nowhere for me to run to or hide away.

It caught me, one of the 200 different types of cancers chose me.

Mr Patel

Official: I was diagnosed with breast cancer on the 5th February 2016, Oh my God!

I stopped all my plans and my life was put on hold. I didn't know what was going to happen.

Apprehensively I attended the first appointment to see Mr Patel. He was the surgeon assigned to perform the surgery and save my life.

He confirmed officially the abnormalities were cancer, stage 1. The cancer type was aggressive, grade 2 intermediate growing. I had invasive lobular breast cancer, apparently this does not always form a lump, it may not show up in mammograms, so it can be difficult to diagnose, under the microscope it may show up as a thickened area of breast tissue rather than a lump.

I had hormone breast cancer, that means that the cancer cells grew in response to the hormone oestrogen. Hormone receptors are proteins, found in and on breast cells, they pick up hormones signals telling the cells to grow.

There are so many forms of cancer, I had to read this over and over again to understand what type I had. I welled up and then just simply cried and cried and cried when it finally sunk in.

It was then that I realised Mr Patel was to stay with me throughout. He was my assigned consultant, the one responsible for getting rid of the cancer, the one to perform a mastectomy. My life was in his blessed hands.

I sat in this all familiar waiting room in the Oncology section. I waited to be called into Mr Patel's consultation room, I thought I was the expert when it came to reading faces, expressions and body language, I looked around for the signs in anticipation. This one defeated me, I was not expecting this. I didn't expect nor could I read my anticipated fate.

'Verna Norton!'

'Yes,' without hesitation with my coat still on my back and bag still firmly on my shoulder I walked to his room with a mission. I bit my tongue so hard I could taste the blood filling up my mouth. I placed myself in the chair, this felt like I was about to be the executed.

Face to face with Mr Patel, with my husband to the right, breast care nurse Alura also stood to the side and remained on her feet. Her role was to act as a mediator.

I thought that I heard cancer!

"Say that again," I asked, something blocked all the words from my mouth from being delivered, they somewhat seemed distorted.

He repeated, "I am afraid it is cancer, I am so sorry." He then looked away, he fixed his gaze to the door behind me.

I looked in amazement, "Say it again please," I demanded, "you said that too quickly, I could not absorb what was being said."

My voice was faint as I became desperate, like being in the firing line pleading for my life to be spared.

The tones in his voice and my vision became distorted. I could no longer hear what he was saying and I could see flowers, loads of flowers as though a funeral was being prepared for me.

Is he messing with my head? Is this some kind of sick joke?

I stood up as I picked up my shoulder bag and placed it on my shoulder.

This feeling of shame threw its blanket over my shoulders, "Don't you dare throw shit on me," I said. "What have I done wrong?" I questioned.

Is this judgement day? Who is going to be my friend? Who is going to help me through this? I felt as though I was slowly losing control, I couldn't grip this one, I was falling to pieces. I felt my insides falling apart and dropped to the cold hard stone floor. Concerned, all three rushed and before I knew it I was back in the chair, like a torture chamber.

"Mr Patel, say that again please," I pleaded.

Mr Patel then looked at breast care nurse Alura as though he was looking for backup. I then knew that I was being placed in the category of not being straightforward. He squinted as he looked at his watch and a frown caused a crease on his forehead, he then repeated this impatiently. I floated out of my body, and observed them from above.

Suddenly I wasn't sure that I wanted to get the answers to my question.

Mr Patel diverted his attention to my husband for any possible signs of movement. Well as far as he was concerned everything he had to say had already been said.

I sat attentively, the spine in my back upright to meet the rigidity of the chair. I wanted and needed more time, I was a virgin at receiving such news, there was no mercy. I felt that I had been shot.

I felt for the loose hair on my head to my left and right of my face that was dangling aimlessly. I reached up with my arms and clasped with both fingers and again raised my arms to motion backwards. This was my absolute desperate attempts to tuck every loose strand of hair behind my ears. I repeated this process several times as I opened my eyes as wide as I could, I was desperate to absorb every word this time, every single word and motion.

I looked deeply into Mr Patel's face for any doubt or hum, but there was none forthcoming. None that I could read as I caught a glimpse of his newly placed dental filling as he spoke. "I am prescribing you Tamoxifen, this will stop the cancer from growing." He scribbled out the prescription before passing it to Nurse Alura.

The tapping of her foot got louder and louder, plainly impatient and busy.

"Mr Patel, please slow down, you said that too fast, again, say it again," I demanded in desperation that this nightmare would end and I would wake from this nightmare.

"Mr Patel, please just tell me one more time," I could feel that I was involuntarily repeating after him. I followed his lips as though I was being taught to speak my first words. I turned and looked at my husband to the right, he too was glued to Mr Patel. It felt as though we were both watching a play intently, suddenly I felt a warm hand grasp into my fingers and entangled in mine.

He refused to make eye contact with me. I looked at Mr Patel and all of a sudden he inherited a stiff flipping neck, he refused to look me in the face as he again fixated his stare to the door behind me, enough was said.

I looked at Nurse Alura, she looked at Mr Patel, it appeared that my reaction was usually unexpected. I felt alone in this small room containing the four of us, I could feel the tears trickle down my face, I couldn't control them, everything was involuntary as I was led out of the room by my husband's firm grip, I can't remember how. I was motionless and became temporarily numb. I am not sure how I ended up in the car on route home.

I hated Mr Patel and Nurse Alura and their cruel delivery of this devastating news.

I felt that it was so well rehearsed. I mean, it was well structured and professional, they were familiar with delivering this type of news and it showed. She told me that she would answer any questions afterwards, again in her efforts to free my chair up for the next patient.

I felt totally helpless and vulnerable.

My 10 minute slot was up, there were other patients waiting, the queue was getting longer and the conveyor belt was moving fast.

Once on this conveyor belt, the green light button was pressed, that was it. I was going through the process.

I questioned my life. What has my existence been about, I asked? Have I done all that I wanted to do? No, I was not ready to wither and die yet.

Telling the Family

Telling my family was one of the hardest things I have ever done in my life.

Thank God it was the weekend, the Friday before Sunday's pole dancing class with my daughter. I didn't get it, what's going on? I can't go pole dancing anymore. I called my daughter on her mobile phone, "Sam," I said sternly, "I cannot attend the pole dancing session with you anymore," I wanted to end the phone call there and then.

I have said what I had to say.

"Oh, why Mum, trust you not to see it through," she joked!

I could hear the disappointment in her voice, "Come on you only have two sessions to go, come on," she said offering encouragement, "don't cop out you've done so well, don't give up now, we are partners and we have a show to perform in three weeks time."

Quick, think, think, think, as the thinking files in my head were working up to a frenzy. I could not tell her like this.

My voice started to creak, "I'm hung over and worse for wear, too much Grey Goose last night."

"Ok, next week, Mum, we will practice the dance, shimmy, shimmy, slide down, peep and up again. Sexy!"

Oh Gosh! I need to tell her the truth, soon, in my own way. How could I shatter this enthusiasm? Why spoil the show? But then I questioned over and over, what's right, what's wrong, why do I want to deliver this bad news to my beautiful daughter, should I go along and keep quiet, but for how long?

What if I make it worse, what if she doesn't forgive me. What am I going to do while I am dying? But then I questioned, why should I lie to her, would she forgive me? These thoughts and doubts, questions and answers went around and around my head for hours tormenting me; it was as though I was going through a maze of mental torture.

I was confused and felt all the emotions at once. I felt heavy and exhausted as I played out all the potential scenarios in my head.

I visualised all the scenarios and accounted for all the potential reactions I would be faced with when I finally told her.

I felt that I had to prepare her fully. I was no further forward, two hours later I was in the same situation facing the same dilemma.

Five days passed, texting was easy. I was tormented everyday... thank God my children no longer lived at home, I could delay delivering this sad news. There were two more days left until we were due to meet up.

Oh my God. What the hell am I going to tell her? Not only that how am I going to tell her?

I practiced and practiced, anticipating disappointment, tears and disbelief. I called her mobile, without asking how she was or how her day was going I blurted out, "Sorry Sam, I can't do pole dancing anymore, so cancel my appointment."

"Why Mum, we only have one more session to go, don't cop out now?"

"Just come around." I said hesitantly, "I need to see you after work."

After work came, it was six forty-five, I felt nauseous for the whole four hours prior.

My mind was working overtime as I pictured dozens of scenarios and potential endings to this absolute nightmare.

I felt as though I was watching a car crash in slow motion.

The pain I felt inside was excruciating.

I paced up and down the kitchen. The moment came and I watched her through the living room window at the front of the house, she walked down the path way without a care in the world. As she walked nearer to the door, I could feel my heart pounding, I felt that I was going to have a heart attack, it echoed within my body.

I opened the door before she could place her key in the lock.

I pounced like a panther, as soon as I caught sight of her beige coat as she came through the door. The dishcloth was still in my hand, due to nerves. It was moulded into a twisted curly pigtail shape.

I could feel the sweat dripping down the back of my neck, my hair was wet, I couldn't take this anymore and got in first... without any further delay.

"Sam?"

"Yes, Mum," as she kicked off her shoes and threw herself backwards she then threw her handbag to the side covered over with her jacket and sank into the sofa. She was home and looking at me.

"Come on then, Mum. What's happening?"

"I won't be going pole dancing anymore," I coughed and felt myself choking, my tonsils decided to block my airway. I can't do this, but I must, I thought. I carried on...

"I have been diagnosed with breast cancer." SILENCE. There, I've said it now... I looked at her and immediately looked away and fixed my stare on a small insect in the corner of the room. I think it was a small beetle, perhaps a queen ant, oh I don't know. I sensed that she was looking at me in disbelief, the silence lasted for what seemed forever...

I was still looking at the insect trying to figure out how it got there, as I inspected further I tried to ascertain what type of insect it was and where it was going to go after the kitchen...

There was silence...

I looked at my daughter, she fixed her stare at me. I could see the signs of disbelief, did she think I was going to break out in laughter, a song or dance perhaps? She didn't move, she was motionless as she looked at me for the go ahead. There was no going ahead, I didn't know where I was going either, I also lost my direction. It felt like an hour...

As her mother, I had to get a grip of this situation and take the lead, how could I deliver such a cruel message without softening the aftercare... It felt as though I sprayed CS gas and would now be required to administer the aftercare and reassurance.

I racked my brain to think about my next move.

"I am so lucky, Sam," I said, the words seemed to echo, "it was caught early, so they can treat it, princess. I am going to be fine and it's all going to be ok, I promise." as I spoke, I knew I was making this pledge to her, I am going to be fine... I looked at her every move.

This was now my mission, I felt desperate in my attempts to justify the delivery of such a brutal blow.

"I promise, I will be okay, I want to see you grow old, I want to see my grandchildren. This is not the end. Grandchildren!"

"Oh, stop it mum."

My mother and my sister came around after an invite to dinner on a Tuesday evening. It was their turn.

I had worked it all out in my head, dinner first then boom! The delivery of the news then the aftercare, reassurance, softener, job done... This went over and over in my head until their arrival.

"Mum, do you fancy coming around on Tuesday about 7pm? I'm cooking dinner and inviting Shirley so we can catch up," unsuspecting mum replied yes, OK.

I then texted my sister; "Shirley, I'm cooking dinner on Tuesday, for about 7pm, fancy popping around? Mum and Sam are going to be there?"

"Yes, would love to," she replied.

"Sam, Nanny and Shirley are coming around for dinner and I am going to tell them, would you come around too? I need your support..."

"Okay, Mum. I'll be there, poor Nanny," she said, "I hope she will be ok..."

"I know, that's why I need you there…"

"I'll be there, Mum."

After our meal, it was about 7pm all three of us sat on the sofa, relaxing. My husband arranged to make himself scarce, everything was going to plan, as the moment came closer.

My heart was beating faster and faster, I was sweating and I couldn't think straight. What if I made my mother ill? What if? What if? What if?

I psyched myself up and felt a sense of inner strength from within, breaking out in a cold sweat at the same time, I could feel the palpitations in my chest as I wiped the sweat away, I felt a sickness of nausea in my stomach, I wanted to vomit through frustration and anticipation.

I could not prolong this agony any longer.

I went into the mode of delivering a death message, I did this many times at work, this was the only way I could cope and detach myself from nightmare reality.

That bit in my throat decided to raise it's ugly head again. It found a way to get trapped in my airways, as the same motions continued blowing into my airways I coughed and almost choked again.

I coughed twice and took a deep breath, in and out, in and out. "Mum! Shirley!" again I could hear myself say Mum the first time around almost like an echo Mum, Shirley.

"Do you remember the time when I told you both that I was going for a mammogram, it was a few weeks ago? Well I had it done, what an experience it was," I watched as my mum listened attentively.

My sister struggled to keep up, I repeated sparingly to check that she understood each point before I went any further, she watched my lips as I spoke slowly, and emphasised my words over pronouncing and maintaining eye contact with both of them to be assured that we were all at the same pace.

"The tests revealed that I have early stage breast cancer," confident that I said it once, I repeated it again, it felt like my speech had reverted into slow motion... I have been diagnosed with breast cancer.

I noticed my mother looking down towards her chest, then she looked at me. I looked at my sister and over pronounced the words, BREAST CANCER. I touched her arm and stroked it gently, I consciously spoke slowly and clearly, she confirmed that she understood, I then placed my hand on my chest to emphasis where it had been located.

She looked at me and repeated after me, "You have breast cancer." Relieved that she understood this time, I reaffirmed yes.

I opened both hands and as a gesture of greeting, I said, "Yes, Yes," as I placed them across my chest as protection. "Yes."

Mum was silent, it was almost as though I had shot her, she was shocked and did not move.

Before my very eyes, I could see my mum's world was crumbling, life was unfair, not her baby. I could see the sorrow and helplessness, what could she do to take this pain away? There were no plasters or pain killers to administer? No bush or medicines could solve this one, it took a further five minutes of emotional turmoil, pain and predictions, all in one.

Whilst I was waiting for mum to digest this devastating news, I felt guilty, how dare I bring this news to upset her so? It was

as though I was a child bringing home a bad school report. How could I be so cruel and bring shame on the family? This illness was a taboo no one dared to entertain, cancer the plague of the earth.

Once this cruel message had sunk in the emotions and thoughts were recycled and processed, tears took hold and she cried uncontrollably.

This was painful and heartbreaking to witness and I caused it, I was to blame. Mum looked in disbelief as she listened and watched my every move; it was almost as though she disappeared out of her soul temporarily.

I hope to bring comfort to those feeling alone in the face of breast cancer.

My sister's deafness added to the frustrations and emotions whilst trying to deliver the information.

At the best of times the translation and response to a single question took minutes.

And even that's before those tricky vocabulary questions such as, 'what's a mammogram,' or even 'what's a hospice?'

I understand that there may be no equivalent sign in ASL. There would be in that case a lot of finger spelling, and a lot of 'what do you mean?' and 'give me an example' and back and forth.

I wonder how the healthcare professionals prepare for this?

Writing this book for these different audiences was difficult; people speaking different languages, with different hearing abilities, disabilities and different cultures.

After a short while the message was absorbed like a sponge thrown into water, silence seeped in and within a short while turned into uncontrollable sobbing.

Mum looked at me, her eyes filled with water, "You can't go before me, I'll go…"

Oh my god, she thinks that I am going to die.

"Mum, we cannot negotiate, the higher being has called for me, Mum. We cannot choose, we cannot volunteer or nominate."

I've done it, I thought to myself, there is no turning back now. They both know, my mum and sister have now been told. I can now move forward from this hurdle. What a hard task, thank goodness the emotions are now a thing of the past, they can now help me through this process of dealing with this sentence.

Surprisingly I did not get the reaction I expected from my sister. She was strong and controlled and very matter of fact, this in itself confirmed to me that everything was going to be ok.

My son. Here we go again. I insisted that he would receive message from me and me only… in person.

I called his mobile "Alex, when are you home?"

"This weekend mum, Why?"

"Nah just wondering."

The weekend came, I could not sleep the night before. I felt sick in my stomach as it churned with unsettled emotions, hurt and guilt.

In frustration, I paced up and down as again I rehearsed several potential scenarios and situations pre-empting how he may react. I went through at least six scenarios and adapted my voice to ensure that this message I was about to deliver would be as palatable as possible.

I chopped and changed to perfection, I wanted this process to be as smooth as possible.

As I waited over night for the boy to arrive from his three-hour journey from the Westcountry, I waited in desperation as I practiced and rehearsed how I was going to deliver the news, my news.

Alex arrived with his bag and I observed like an out of body experience.

He kissed me as I opened the door to save him using his keys, his usual kiss on the cheek as he took his bag upstairs.

It felt like forever as I waited for him to come back downstairs, I paced up and down, up and down in the living room. A reminder of waiting for the pregnancy results and seeing that strip turn blue for positive.

His heavy footsteps came thumping down the staircase.

I couldn't wait for him to get something to eat or arrange any plans with his mates without delivering this news.

"Alex! I need to let you know that I have been diagnosed with early stage breast cancer."

I waited for his reaction as he looked at me and plonked himself down on the sofa.

"Really, Mum?" he said in disbelief, I don't know what he was thinking, I couldn't read this one. Perplexed, he did not question me and took my word for it.

I continued my impassive expressions.

I could hear voices in my head filling in the gaps... you are not joking? I then to myself he would ask if there were any doubts and why would I joke or exaggerate about such thing.

I then tried to think what he may have been thinking, while the silence took its course.

He is my son, I am his mother, he needs be to be around right now, I was not ready to die, what was I going to do about it then, what is the plan, what did I have in place to reassure him and prove that I was going to be ok?

I have always been in control and I was not going to let this one beat me. He needs his mother around.

I went on autopilot almost as though I was being restarted from within like a dying battery being recharged.

Thank God I was back on track, back in control. I replied, "Well," I said confidently, "I am having all the tests, but it was caught very early therefore I am going to be ok, I promise. Shall we book some holiday breaks for when this is all over?" I said apprehensively.

In disbelief, but admiration, he looked at me, his eyes told me that he was somewhat confused, our eyes met and we both smiled together before getting out our iPads. We booked a short break in Norfolk to recuperate by the seaside.

I knew that I was going to be ok, I had to be. That mother instinct kicked in. I then felt a different type of inner strength, it felt like I was drowning but fighting to keep my head above the water...

Children, the sentiments were felt wholeheartedly. You will rely on your mother's strength until her dying day. I will be back in your lives. I wanted to go with you when you left me at the Hospital bedside, inside I was screaming, don't leave me here, I want to be back in life, I want to be included with the living, but my stability was being ripped away. I didn't want this, I was being confronted with making one of the hardest decisions. A life or death situation.

The rest of my family and friends were then informed of my illness in a sort of order of preference and priority. I didn't want to lose control of this simple task and it was for me to dictate and reveal the extent of my illness. It was clear that I was fragile, but I was told by my close family that I was going to be ok.

My daughter looked at me and kissed my forehead as she said, "Goodbye, Mum I will pray for you."

Wow! I thought, she is going to pray for me. She was never religious and she is going to pray for me! Gosh I thought... Things are bad. I would like to be a fly on the wall, I wonder what she said?

I think that I actually inherited a sixth sense and that my hearing had improved remarkably.

I could hear the conversations my husband would have with his friends and relatives, he would discuss my treatment and the state of my health.

I could overhear conversations of my husband being quizzed about the stages, the lymph node and the spread of the disease.

I couldn't quite make out whether it was of genuine concern or sheer nosiness. I could feel my blood boiling with anger and the frustrations of my own personal health being shared with all and sundry. Sympathy is very nice, but not an excuse for burdens of your own misgivings to be confused and entangled with my own battle.

I would often challenge this and question when and at what point did I employ a spokesperson.

What right did people feel they had to discuss my business? Why the sudden interest in my personal health?

I couldn't understand why folk wanted to know the ins and outs of my illness, some would ring to glean information, so painfully sad. I was intrigued by the sudden medical expertise and knowledge that was obtained overnight by folk. Now this was what I called a flipping miracle.

I was bombarded with, 'Well Sheila had cancer and she did this and that…' and 'Brenda passed away because it went to her lymph nodes' and 'Ethel down the road had cancer and died, she kept her, illness quiet' and blah, blah, blah…

Nosey, nosey and nosey… Why did I not generate the same level of interest whilst I was fit, healthy and fly?

Sensitivity kicked in, I would hear laughter, I would look around and ask why are you laughing?

Are you laughing at me, who are you messaging on your mobile, is it about me?

How can the rest of the world be so happy while I am dying inside? It was then I felt the hood of loneliness draping over my soul, despite being in a room of people. I was so lonely.

I had to give up on this weary wasted energy, because I would need all of my strength to face this battle set before me.

Bravery prevailed as I carried on regardless, adapting an initially quivering lip before developing a stiff upper lip approach.

I felt great pain and hurt for what I was being put through, it felt as though I was the one chosen to walk the walk of burden, this disease within my soul needed to come out. I had no control, I had to wait my turn, wait for the processes and procedures to take place. After all, I was not the only one.

I saved the mourn-mongers from joining me in reliving my journey of this disease, the pain and uncertainty of not knowing what was going to happen next.

I don't feel that I have robbed you of the grieving process, I have simply spared your energy for another occasion.

I would often see the look of pity in their eyes. They would widen, filled with pity and predictions. I could see looks of fear in their eyes. It felt almost as though I was due to be taken away to the dog rescue home like an unwanted puppy, I would often catch folk staring thinking I was unaware.

I caught you looking for the signs of decay, inspecting my hair as I flicked it to one side.

Was this ugly to take its toll on me now?

I caught the eyes of those who would look me in the eyes for signs of last night's tears, inspect my face for the process to excel. My teeth for premature decay and general viable signs of this grave illness' cape of death.

My family would visit my bedside with love, fuss and concern, the conversations and laughter would flow. I wanted to leave with them, I did not want to stay in the hospital ward. It was punishing. When they left I was alone again, they took the laughter and joy with them, it felt that they had come to my funeral and then left me to fend for myself alone in the grave. I felt as though I was being buried alive.

I was ahead of this game. Nope, I said to myself, I am not ready for this, I am not accepting this expected decay at all. The grooming process was stepped up a few notches.

The next day I went into a local DIY shop and selected colour swatches. I then certified myself as a personal shopper; I had the tools to self-analyse compatible colours.

Hairstylist Monday. Chiropodist Tuesday. Brazilian wax Wednesday. Shellac manicure and pedicure on Thursday. Dentist and Eye test Friday. Clothes shopping and lunch Saturday.

Rest on Sunday, that's more like it.

Folk would often say, 'Cor you look well, considering...'

Of course I do, what the hell did you expect?

The Tests

1. Physical examinations.
   This was to check for signs of the disease, lumps and anything unusual.
   Clinical Breast Exam;
   Doctors and surgeons carefully felt the breasts and underarms. In the early stages I remember staring at the ceilings, wishing I was somewhere else instead.
2. Mammogram.
   X-ray of the breast between two plates used to take pictures of the breast tissue. This was painful, my breasts were squashed into these plates and this experience was surreal. This is where the cause for concern started.
   Ultra sound, a high energy magnet with sound waves, the computer made tunes which saw the new lumps forming.
3. MRI.
   Magnetic radio waves to make a series of detailed pictures of both breasts.
4. Blood Chemistry.
   Blood sample is checked to measure the amounts of certain substances released into the blood by organs and tissues.
5. Biopsy.
   The removal of cells and tissues so that they can be viewed under the microscope by a pathologist for signs of cancer.
   I had the core biopsy, the removal of tissue using a wide needle.
   Then a fine needle aspiration the removal of tissue using a thin needle.

Sentinel lymph node biopsy, a radioactive substance and blue dye is injected near the tumour to detect any spread of the disease.

6. Angiogram.

An image like a scan, this shows the blood vessels, and indicates how well the heart is pumping blood prior to the DIEP surgery.

7. Mastectomy.

The medical term for the surgical removal of one or both breasts, partially or completely. A mastectomy is usually carried out to treat breast cancer.

8. Reconstruction.

Breast reconstruction can be done at different times, depending on what works best for individuals.

All the work is done in one operation, you wake up with a rebuilt breast, however this may not be possible for those who require Radiotherapy or Chemotherapy.

9. DIEP Flap Surgery.

A muscle and skin sparing surgery. Fat, skin and blood vessels are cut from the wall of the lower belly and moved up to your chest to rebuild your breast.

Your stomach is then tucked flat and your breast is filled with your own body fat.

Every week I felt like a guinea pig on an experimental treadmill. I felt as though I had become an exhibit for all of the tests. I kept reassured and repeatedly told myself that this was to make me better. My body became detached as I reluctantly succumbed and gave in to this experiment, like a whore forced to engage a punter. It was not them that I saw when I fantasised. I hated the injections, I hated blood tests, I hated all the intrusions of the spiteful needles. The nurses and doctors would miss a vein and often accidentally intrude on my bone, painful, very painful, I hated that too.

I would often find myself asking time and time again, what did I do so wrong to deserve this?

Polish Sisters

It was a Thursday evening, 15.05 exactly. I was going to be late to my appointment with Octavia. I pressed on and eventually got there seconds before the time. When I approached the glass door, I saw Octavia preparing her chair for me, her next client. I went into the store and she kissed me on the cheek, "It's great to see you."

"You, too," I repaid the compliment almost immediately. "It is so good to see you, you look amazing." I went to add, "Octavia…"

"Yes, Verna? What is it…?"

I really wanted to say, but could not. I do not feel that I am brave enough and mentally strong enough to experience all the pain that I'm going through. I certainly did not want her pity either. "Now listen to me, princess, you are going to do my microdermabrasion and basic manicure and pedicure, I'll have a clear gloss please."

"Oh," she said, surprised that I did not want a normal bright red shellac.

"No, not this time. I'll be leaving for a while, so will be side-lined for about a month or so."

"Why?" she asked carefully, "then leave?"

"I'm… having a boob job and tummy tuck," as I said it I felt I was once again coming alive. I suddenly felt a breath of excitement, "so I have a flat stomach and lift my breasts. They are too flat." I waited for her reaction.

Our eyes met, full of emotion she raised her hands to the side when he grabbed me with both hands, there was no escape, she looked at me, face to face, and said: "Oh my God. You're going to have a boob job and a tummy tuck? It is nice, I want it too. In my country we have beautiful women, I want that, as you say in English, the works," she went on to say, "I want it too."

"You just have to save."

Full of emotion, she then raised her top and said, "Look," then leaned forwards with her breasts with her hand, "I want, I want."

Our eyes met, as we laughed.

"You're so brave," she said, she then focused on the water and cotton ready for my treatment.

"I want it for me, too."

She then started the procedure as she gently lifted my face and stroked it with the flannel gently stroking before the sounds of the microdermabrasion needle started to buzz and then went on to do the procedure, I felt as though my face was gently being filed.

"I do nails red? Do your…"

Before I could answer that she went on to say, "I'll manicure nails nicely with bright red, Yes?"

She looked at me for an answer.

"OK, OK Octavia," I did not want to tell her that I had to be naked for my next cancer treatments.

"Make sure you come and show me, when you do all of this. I am so excited for you, I also want it too. How much will it cost you?"

"Oh around six thousand," I blurted out. "Oh, I'm not sure how much exactly, my husband is treating me." I looked at her, I wondered if she could see that I was fibbing.

She replied, "All I can say is that it is a lot of money in Poland too. Awww beautiful," she said in admiration, her face beamed in approval like the sunlight.

Well that's blown my chances of going to heaven... Thank you Octavia, you inspired me, I felt whole again.

To my beautiful Polish sisters, welcome.

Byl czwartek dokladnie godzina 15.05. Spoznie sie na wizyte u Oktawii. Pospieszylam sie jednak i udalo mi sie zdazyc na czas. Kiedy dotarlam do szklanych drzwi, zobaczylam,ze Oktawia szykowala juz krzeslo dla nastepnej klientki, dla mnie. Weszlam do salonu i ona ucalowala mnie w policzek mowiac "Wspaniale Cie znow widziec".

"Ciebie rowniez "odpowiedzialam. "Dobrze cie widziec, wygladasz wspaniale "po czym zaczelam mowic dalej "Oktawia..."

Tak Verna ? O co chodzi?

Naprawde chcialam jej powiedziec ale nie moglam sie zdobyc na to. Nie czulam sie na tyle odwazna, na tyle silna psychicznie zeby przezyc ten bol ponownie mowiac o tym. Nie chcialam zdecydowanie tez jej litosci.

-Sluchaj ksiezniczko zrob mi mikrodermabrazje i zwykly manicure razem z pedicure, poprosze o przezroczysty lakier tylko.

-Oh -odpowiedziala tylko Oktawia zdziwiona,ze poprosilam o przezroczysty lakier zamiast tak jak zawsze o czerwone zelowe paznokcie.

-Dlaczego tylko przezroczysty?

-Nie, nie tym razem. Nie bedzie mnie przez jakis czas, nie bede mogla umowic sie na kolejna wizyte przez jakis miesiac albo dluzej.

-Dlaczego? Nie bedziesz juz wiecej przychodzic? Opuszczasz mnie?

-"Bede...bede miala operacje plastyczna piersi i brzucha. "Po tym jak to wypowiedzialam poczulam jakbym wracala do zycia wreszcie. Poczulam nagly przyplyw energii "bede miala plaski brzuch I podniesione piersi. Sa zbyt obwisle." Czekalam na jej reakcje.

Nasz wzrok sie spotkal. Podekscytowana zlapala mnie za boki i zajrzala mi w oczy mowiac "O Boze. Bedziesz miala operacje plastyczna piersi i brzucha?! Ale fajnie, ja tez bym chciala. W moim kraju sa piekne kobiety wiesz. Ja tez bym chciala miec -jak to Wy Angielki mowicie- taka robote zrobiona. Tez bym tak chciala.

-"Musisz tylko oszczedzic na to" powiedzialam.

Rozemocjonowana Oktawia podniosla do gory bluzke i krzyknela "Zobacz!"-obejmujac dlonmi swoje piersi- "Ja tez chce, ja tez chce"

Popatrzylysmy sobie w oczy i wybuchnelysmy smiechem.

53

-"Jestes bardzo odwazna" powiedziala Oktawia i skupila sie na szykowaniu wody i narzedzi do zabiegu. "Tez bym tak chciala" dodala i zaczela delikatnie obmywac moja twarz flanelowa chusta zanim przystapila do mikrodermobrazji. Slyszalam brzeczenie igly i czulam jak moja twarz ozywa.

Oktawia zapytala ponownie czy ma zrobic mi paznokcie na czerwono i zanim zdazylam odpowiedziec jej, szybko dodala "Zrobie paznokcie ladnie na czerwono jak zawsze dobrze?" "

Zgodzilam sie.Nie chcialam jej mowic,ze do kolejnego etapu, operacji na raka bede musiala byc naga i bez makijazu.

- Przyjdz i pokaz mi jak bedziesz juz po operacji plastycznej. Jestem bardzo ciekawa I ciesze sie, ze bedziesz ja miala. Ja tez chce to zrobic. Ile to bedzie cie kosztowac?

-Okolo szesciu tysiecy. Nie jestem dokladnie pewna bo to prezent od meza i on za to placi.

Popatrzylam na nia i sie zastanawialam czy zauwazyla, ze drgalam.

Oktawia odpowiedziala-"Jedno co moge powiedziec to to,ze taki zabieg kosztuje bardzo duzo pieniedzy w Polsce rowniez."Jej twarz byla rozpromieniona.

No trudno. Moje szanse na pojscie do nieba przelecialy.

Dziekuje Ci Oktawio, ze mnie tak napelnilas radoscia i sprawilas,ze znow poczulam ze zyje.

Mojej pieknej polskiej siostrze- wyrazy szacunku.

Breaking the news to work colleagues.

"Girls, boys. Amanda, Lottie, Eleanor, Helen, Jatinder, Ioona, Baljit, Piotr, Lee, James, Richard, will you all join me in the conference room please? It won't take long," this was said officially, the message and urgency was in my voice.

I looked at the big noisy clock on the wall. It was 11am. Piotr looked up adjusting his glasses, pushing them back to the bridge of his nose. I looked at the hefty paperwork before him, it was clear that this had better be urgent. Why would I demand his time in such a manner?

The rest of my colleagues gathered in the conference room, they looked at each other with blank expressions on their faces, I could hear the whispersssssss...

"I wonder what this is about?" I overhead Baljit question Ioona.

"I bet it's that Griefy case going to court."

I could see the look of intrigue, why would I call you all in... I took centre court and opened my stage as they found seats within this compact room, last used for the early morning management meetings daily at 9am.

"Er...Well I have bought you in here to tell you that I have been diagnosed with early stage breast cancer."

"Oh my God. Not you as well," roared Helen, "for fucks sake, first Kitty and now you!"

Kitty was also the driving force for pursuing my mammogram. DI Kitty Lou was diagnosed with breast cancer six months prior. That was a shock and now me, what the hell is going on.

I said the words so quickly, there was no room for digestion or preparation for the quick severity of the words. Silence filled the room, I tried to look at each person eye to eye, I wanted to engage and make this as personal as possible. I couldn't see but heard Amanda sob, she could not belief what she was hearing, why would I say such a cruel thing to hurt her, she was my friend. She then started to cry uncontrollably.

"Don't cry, I am going to be fine," as I looked around the room again, I could see the anticipation in the others waiting patiently for the next word, it appeared that I took centre stage and I had to hold my audience.

The look of disbelief filled the room as I looked at every one of them.

I could see the question being raised silently, what type of announcement is this?

Is this normal, who with cancer says or makes an announcement like this... What else should I have said? Shying away would only amplify the stigma, how else am I to put it? The BIG C, the C WORD or the SILENT KILLER.

I then felt a sense of peace and relief, I was relaxed and felt comfortable, this part was out of the way, "I have been diagnosed with early stage breast cancer and will be undergoing treatment," I repeated.

The look of disbelief, shock, disgust, filled the room like someone had filled it with smoke ready to set the ambience of a disco. I could hear the echoes of a sick joke and then the words appeared superficially on the ceiling, Nightmare, Wicked, Sick Joke, Wake Up, Bad Dream. I was bedazzled with these words as I sought solace from looking up at the ceiling for strength. They were floating around... Cancer... Sickness... Stop Now... Games... Seriousness... as I was lost in the words that appeared I heard the soft voice of Charlotte who spoke first. Her voice was choked as she struggled for an answer on behalf of the team.

"When did this happen? You don't look like it, Vern, you look really well?"

"Erm," I said, doubtfully, lost for words. I asked myself, what the hell was I to look like, myself? No I want to look like me and I was determined to beat this wicked, wicked, cruel disease.

I walked around the room, almost as though I miraculously appeared in a university lecture with this audience, I began to tell my story as I started to relive the very day I was prompted to get a mammogram.

Within seconds Dora hit the floor, I thought that she was having a fit, she rolled around the carpet and was sobbing and repeatedly said, "No, no, no."

What the hell I thought, I hardly know her.

As Ioona helped her up, she cried, "That's so awful."

I wondered if she was crying for me or someone else, I hardly knew her. Ironically, I think it was her first week at the station.

People associate you with illness and then if you get angry or upset they say it's the cancer, when it is nothing to do with that.

I returned to my computer terminal for the last time and set my out of office until further notice.

There was a warm sense of smugness. No more work for a little while, finalisation. That's me done for a little while, from here on, a new chapter of the unknown. I still thought to myself secretly, will I die?

I went into reflection mode and I was suddenly taken back there and I could actually smell the room of sterility. I repeated the prognosis. You have Cancer! My voice changed, this was no joke, it was a warning message. Go and get checked out.

Don't wait for a lump alone, check for signs, if in doubt get checked out, the earlier the better... I consider myself to be lucky... be lucky yourselves. It's no secret and it's nothing to be ashamed about.

You have all heard it from me yourselves, I've told you from my mouth, whatever the rumours are to follow from this day on, this is my real account.

Aggression and anger, if I could have visited myself in hospital I would have said to myself everything was going to be ok, joy and courage, fearless maybe, I choose life!

They gave me letters, four different hospitals for my treatments. The whole of the summer was spent travelling to different flipping hospitals.

I was so tired and sick and just wanted to get home as soon as possible.

It affects the entire family. I would often be asked, 'What are you doing tomorrow?' My diary would be filled with hospital appointments, often a 100 mile round trip.

The parking tickets, the packed lunches, the coins ready to feed the ticket machine.

The long days waiting around in the waiting rooms. It was so emotionally draining.

Was this the temporary stop before the restart of life?

The night before

I was in my favourite hide out, La Sala, Chigwell, enjoying a meal, a glass of wine and oh a cheeky porn star martini of course. I was not sure if this was to be my last... but I was well enough to go out and socialise. I toasted to the future as the freeing of my soul from cancer was about to begin. Apprehensive, but little did I know what I was about to face.

My journey of pre-treatments and tests had stopped. It was operation time, the big one. I now know that this was just temporary.

This was the night before admission was coming closer. What would be left, I questioned? What state would I be in? Would I be a changed person? These thoughts went around and around my mind like a carousel.

Let Aeki leap into your life, open up your curtains to love and be loved.

I hope this helps you to keep inspired.

Let me be your hero.

Monday! I was not making love by Wednesday... but certainly chilled on Sunday with my last porn star martini before my journey.

Craig, I was also 'Born to do it.'

60

A night with Dusky Dawn

I walked and pondered apprehensively towards the receptionist. I thought to myself I really like this hospital, I felt that there was a great sense of calm in the atmosphere and civility amongst the passer-by.

I waited my turn in this short queue of two persons in front.

"Next, please," said the efficient voice.

Our eyes met, greeting me was this pretty young lady with auburn hair as she pushed her fringe from her eyes she said, "How can I help you."

"I have an appointment with Mr Griffiths at 3pm."

She looked at me with approval, I think it's because I quickly identified her name. I followed her eyes as they wondered to the pages on the screen in front of her and stopped, I presume, at my details.

"Oh Ok. Turn to the right then down the corridor, bay B."

"Thank you, Emma," I said, she knew that I liked her through the tone of my voice.

She replied, "I like your eyelashes." See, I may have been a cancer patient then, but all was not lost, I thought to myself as I took a sudden bounce in my step. I was walking tall.

With Dave by my side I followed the instructions and walked into the waiting room. Of course I would cause some attention; I was the only black female there.

The other patients looked me up and down discreetly. I could feel the curiosity and the looks at the side of my eyes, I would often catch a stray eye that forgot to look away in time, this was met with a sweet acknowledgement.

I grabbed a magazine and admired the clothes and fashion. This is going to be me again, I affirmed and repeated to myself.

I practiced what my new model pout was going to look like, as I discreetly took my mobile phone out, placed it on silent and took a selfie.

The feng shui in me wanted to be comfortably seated, so I moved to the seat facing the white door with my back against the wall. I could see the white door that clearly said 'Mr Griffiths'.

I was able to see every movement of the opening and shutting.

After a while the door took on a life of its own. In went the nurse, then another, then the patient, then another nurse, then another nurse would come out and walk down the corridor, then the patient would exit.

Mixed emotions and hard to read recipients of news were entering and exiting.

I then realised that there was nowhere to cry.

Fuming, it's been three flipping hours, I hissed. As I tutted, the roof of my gum met my tongue and clicked, in disapproval.

Four hours later, "Mrs Norton," I looked up and saw a nurse. My name was next on the list she had cradled in her arms.

"Yes," as I got up eagerly to learn my fate, I grabbed my coat and bag and placed the magazine down on the table full of magazines for the next person.

Ms Dusky Dawn, the other lady also got up.

I looked at her and she looked at me.

"Well, it's just you and me kid." I said in a matter of fact manner

"What your name? My name is Verna."

"Dusky." She replied.

Silence filled the pause as we looked each other up and down. She was wearing a pink T-Shirt and white jeans and green and white training shoes with a red stripe.

I looked down to my shiny stilettos, I caught a glimmer of my face.

We both wore different shoes, but were on the same path...

Myself and Dawn were the only two left. The others were asked to go home and return in the morning due to the lack of beds. We were both led through the double doors to another day ward, two beds reserved for us. The nurse picked up a few hospital robes and walked us through to the ward. She then closed the door behind her and told me that I'd have to take everything off and wear just the robe. She then told me the best way to tie the robe to avoid any embarrassing buttock flash.

"Ward Sister, Ella. May I ask, are we definitely staying here the night to have the operation tomorrow? I don't feel that this can be delayed, I am mentally prepared now."

Little did she know that I had already rehearsed all the reasons why I was not going home that night.

Nurse Ella simply said, "Yes of course you are both staying," no rhyme or reasons or explanations given. Surprised, I looked around before discreetly placing my justification note safely in my pocket.

Ella looked me directly in the face as our eyes meet, we spoke the same language and it was quickly identified that we shared the same humour. It was as though we had met before, she spoke to me as though she knew me. Yep, she had certainly met my type before.

She firmly inserted my confirmation to admissions by a jab to the thigh and issued my fit all size granny DVT green stockings. My reservation to seven days in OXO cube ward was confirmed. I secretly smiled to myself; this was the first stage to be treated.

Due to shortages of beds, Dusky and I were placed on trolleys in the day ward, we didn't care, I think we both felt ready for the sacrifice.

Me and Dusky were chosen together.

I could hear male voices down the end of the corridor.

Oh my GOD, MAN! A male voice.

"Nurse Carol," I joked, "I hope there is no frisky people in the ward, I have not got the energy tonight."

"It's not them, it's you we are worried about," Laughs! They know about me.

Welcoming from the start...

Nurse Carol came around, I felt a sense of calm and compassion in this environment, the choice of menus was plentiful and of good quality. My sincere gratitude for the good old NHS, it was appreciated.

It's was then that I felt within my soul a powerfully great sense of love and appreciation to its highest level.

For manners, I allowed Dusky to choose from the menu first. The bugger chose the last flipping beef lasagne. She quickly learned the etiquette and allowed me to choose the jam sponge and ice cream, that was the last one. We were now even.

We both shared our stories of how our we discovered the breast cancer, we silently and spiritually put each other at ease. Dusky revealed that exactly a year ago she had a hysterectomy.

"What the fuck," I laughed inappropriately, desperately trying to contain myself by placing my hand to cover my mouth and a hand over my fat belly to drown and muzzle some of the laughter, she went on to say in a matter of fact tone, "Verna, if I was to go under an X-ray there would be blank shadows."

Oh my god! I pictured this image in my twisted warped mind. I fixed my eyes to the ceiling and fixated for a second, but she read my actions and we laughed hysterically together until I could hear her soft tones peacefully breathing as she fell into a deep sleep. I think it was at this point we both spiritually became sisters together on this purposeful journey of the unknown.

"Night, Dusky," I whispered.

Within seconds she replied hesitantly, "Good night, Verna, tomorrow is our big day."

Let me play with your body, baby

It was approximately 7am, I was excited for the unknown. I braced myself for the preparations for the forthcoming big operation, I felt scared and excited both at the same time. I had to pinch myself to acknowledge what was actually happening.

Dr Julie came to my bedside, she was one of the surgeons responsible for the reconstruction. She pulled out her black marker and drew on my breast; up and down she swished the pen confidently up the top of my torso, this was an indication of how the immediate mastectomy was to take form.

I took an instant liking to Julie, so was very pretty, with her dark brown hair, dark eyes and half mixed English/Chinese appearance and I could feel that she was going to share her beauty with me as she drew with the ink marker with passion. I felt as though a new sculpture was being formed.

"Dr Julie, could I please have my breast size remain please? Oh and could I have a small 32 inch waist so that it compliments my butt size…"

Acknowledging my request, she smiled sweetly; I could see the expressions on her face filled with great sympathy that beamed from her eyes, sympathy towards me, this nutter ordering a new body. Perhaps this was a type of coping mechanism, which I was totally unaware of, or maybe it was me being vain…

Immediately a stern voice in my head shocked me to reality, 'You are here because actually you have breast cancer, you are going to have a mastectomy and a DIEP flap immediate reconstruction. Got it?'

Next thing some one pushed me forward from behind.

Before I had a chance to see who it was to 'cuss their arse' it was too late as I held on to dear life. It was too late... I was there... deep in the unknown... as I fastened my seat belt the roller coaster ride was to begin.

In my gown, lying face down I was wheeled into the operating theatre, "No, I don't want to go." Was this the end, was I about to face death, I asked?

I remember being wheeled on the trolley, various faces with masks were looking down on me, I felt one of them reach for my wrist and in went the intravenous, right on the wrist bone,

"Please, please would you look after me," I pleaded, I felt scared and naked. "Please look after me," as I gripped an arm of one of the anaesthetists. Slowly reaching down to her right hand, as I gripped tighter I said, "Hold my hand," before I could say "what the Fuck," that was it.

"My name is Laura." She said softly, "everything is going to be ok."

I could hear voices in the background, "You are going to be ok. You are going to be ok." This was being repeated until these words were replaced by echoes fading away in the background."

I was led to a place that I had never been before. I later learned that I lost seven hours of my life.

I came around slowly and peacefully as though I were born again, I was exhausted and filled to the gunnels with wiring and drips.

I woke up slowly, like a gerbil waking from hibernation. I was determined to live to the full. This was my second chance, if I had not already, life to the full this time around, I repeated to myself.

After a short while, I felt anxious, I couldn't move freely as I wanted to. My arms were in pain almost as though I was placed in some sort of crucified position. The pain underneath was unbearable, one arm I could understand but both baffled me, I was restricted in my legs which were bound into a pumping machine, I felt my nose and felt a tube…

"What is this in my nose?" I asked in desperation and curiosity. "What has happened to me? Who put me on the cross?" I shouted.

My arms were aching underneath both arms, was I actually crucified? I know it's Easter, but for God's sake why have I been chosen to be sacrificed, I wondered. Who the hell was it that pushed me off the earth then? Come on, own up?

I must have dozed in and out of consciousness as it all seem to be such a blur after that.

I sat on the edge of my bed, overwhelmed by all the uncertainty and turmoil, I know it's Easter but I think that I was the one that was crucified and placed on the cross, I had actually been unconscious for seven hours.

When I think back now, I cringe at the thought of being an operating object for that whole period of time a whole day virtually…

A short while later I was settled into a side cubicle…

"Hello Verna," I thought the voice was familiar but I could not place where it was from. As I peered over to my right side,

I could see Dusky's statue. It's Dusky! Again reunited to my right.

"Hello, darling. How are you? We've done it. Haven't we done it?"

I could feel my body and soul filling up with joy and gratitude. We are cancer free, I thought that was it... Operation over, the cancer had been cut out. Job done... little did we know that was not officially the all clear. This was just the starting point.

* * *

A sigh of relief and sense of achievement was prevalent. If I could reach up to do a fist punch I would. Due to the pain I settle for a finger wiggle...

I then went into a daze.

"Verna, Verna!" There were hands shaking me, pulling me awake.

"Verna, I am going to need you to wake up, love. Verna."

I feel fingers pulling at my eyelids and a light, blinding bright, shining in.

"Ow!" I blink and pull back, and a hand lets go of my chin.

"Sorry, love, are you OK? Are you awake now?"

The face is disconcertingly close, her eyes staring into mine. I blink again and then nod, "Yes. Yes I am awake."

I don't know when I dozed off.

69

But the closer things get to – to whatever happened, the hazier they get. "What happened? Why am I here?"

I must have spoken the last words aloud for the nurse gives a kindly smile.

"You have had a mastectomy and reconstruction, my love."

"Am I OK?"

"Yes, nothing broken." She has a pleasant Northern accent.

"I have had to wake you. We have to do observations every few hours, just to make sure you've not had a funny turn."

"I was asleep," I say stupidly, and then rub my face, it hurts. I could not raise my arms it was so heavy.

"Careful now," the nurse says. "You've got a few cuts and bruises."

I feel disgusting. I need a pee.

"Can I have a shower?" I ask. My head feels bleary.

The nurse looks down on the chart at the foot of the bed.

She turns and goes, and I catch sight of the silhouette outside the door, the door flapping behind her with a gust of food smells and sounds from outside the corridor.

There was a sense of calm after the storm as I lowered my chin, as I looked down and slowly inspected my state. I looked left side and squealed. I was on a drip and winced at another tube feeding me. I slowly looked down, my feet were wrapped up in a pumping machine. It was very noisy. It was almost as though both legs were in a vacuum being pumped, then as I gently moved my eyes to the right, my now bad arm, where I had the operation was cushioned with folded towels and padding and dressing.

What the hell is going on, I asked myself. What has happened to me? This whole damn thing is so surreal as I gently shook my head in disbelief and raised my eyes up to the Gods.

I noted that I was on the end bay of this four-bed hospital ward called Oxo Cube ward Intensive Care Unit. I quickly learned that I was classed as a high dependency. Yes, effectively intensive care, I repeated to myself.

The team involved in my operation came to see me on an individual basis regularly, this made me feel very special. I felt like they came to check on me and their masterful craftsmanship. They huddled around my bed.

Dr Julie was the first.

"What has happened to me? Have you called Dave? What time is it?" I did not draw breath, but somehow she managed to absorb this lumpy request.

"Well Verna, you have just undergone a seven hour operation. We reconstructed your breast from your stomach and then we decided to move you vein from your neck to your breast area. We felt that this is very strong and able to pump and function effectively."

"We have then tucked your stomach up neatly."

I looked at her wide-eyed in disbelief. This is a fucking miracle! "Thank you. Thank you so much for making me better..."

After a short time, Mr Griffiths the Man came to check on his work as he drew the curtains back. It was our secret. I proudly pulled my top and revealed his work. He smiled with pride at his success.

"Mr Griffiths, oh my God, I can't believe what has happened. Tell me again what have you done." As I focus on his lips to capture every word he repeated word for word what Dr Julie had told me.

In amazement I listened again intensively, if I had access to voice recording this would have definitely been captured. Once this information was finally placed in the filing cabinet in my brain, I said thank you. Wow...

There must have been a meaningful strength in my voice, a sort of affirmation tone, he gleamed as he proudly inspected his work again. He touched and drew with his forefinger how and where, as we discussed, plans for my new belly button and a bit of a nip and tuck after the healing had taken place were necessary.

"Let me be your toy, make me... master." This just blurted out of my mouth, cheeky I know. I don't know what reaction this would have generated, but to be honest, after all I had been through... I was past caring.

Then R Kelly's *let me play with your body baby'* lyrics came to my lips as I sang softly...

Mr Griffiths gently placed the bedding over me to protect his work. I felt that love and proudness beaming as though he had eaten ReadyBrek for breakfast. This was from his soul, he gently tapped the bed in approval and pulled the curtains back.

Sister JoJo then came around and confirmed that the top notches were pleased with my progress as she gently adjusted my legs and said I have just placed your knickers in your side draw for you so that you know where they are... Stop, I didn't know that I had no knickers on.

Oh my God... whilst my legs were akimbo, I was revealing my jewels, especially that one called fanny! Mind you, after what I had been through that was the least of my worries. On reflection it was funny, very funny... I still chuckle with laughter.

As the curtains went back, I noticed two new faces in this dorm of three other beds, Dusky to my right.

Another lady opposite her, who I will refer to as Stella and opposite to me Jeanette.

During the course of the night our eyes met and we politely smiled at each other, intrigued. We knew that we had all been on the same journey.

Both Jeanette and Stella were one day ahead of myself and Dusky. Stella appeared to be in a bad way and there was a lot of commotion coming from her cubicle. Heavy breathing, pumping of the machinery and commotion.

Jeanette's cubicle opposite was calm and peaceful and my new friend Dusky to my right was also calm, but anxious vibes were oozing.

I took a moment to observe this, my new home for the next now six days. I felt at ease and liked where I had been placed and felt safe and secure in this spot.

I had flashbacks and visions taking me back to the first moments of being admitted, whatever happened, whatever was there to put me to the test was now all over. The burden was lifted.

I went down and had the tumour removed at 8am and it is now 4pm, I had lost a day in my life. One whole day, can you believe it? Because I can't.

***

We were together in the ward, the four of us.

We had all undergone the operation; as we quickly synchronised, I learned that I had undergone the longest operation. "Seven hours, seven hours," I repeated in disbelief, "what the hell were they doing to me during this time?" If only I were a fly on the wall!

Jeanette replaced by Candy Pops was moved to another ward, Stella and Dusky...

Candy Pops was not happy, well there was not a lot to be happy about apart from the fact that we were all still alive... as we formed our group, as we began sharing our stories of our pet hates.

"It's the look of pity that does me," says Stella, "It really, really winds me up..."

"Oh no," shouted Dusky, "it's the expertise of some people, all of a sudden they claim to know about your illness." Dusky then raked the hair from her face in confidence.

"No, it's the one where they know how you feel and they know what you are going through. How does that work I ask?" I looked across and noted the nod from Stella in agreement.

"What have I got to show now?" Candy Pops expressed, not particular speaking to anyone in particular...her voice was low and pitiful.

"I can't even look, I have been mutilated. What man is going to want me now?"

"We are cancer free, Candy Pops! Free from cancer. We are the lucky ones..." I replied in my efforts to offer some sort of reassurance, "It could be so much worse, couldn't it?"

I heard a whimper, as I looked up I could see tears rolling from Candy Pops cheeks.

"Candy," I shouted, "Candy babes..." I reached out with my arms but I couldn't get up because I was shackled to the bed and my legs were so heavy with the weight of the cuffed compressions, I was certainly not strong enough, but shouted across the bed opposite. "Candy Pops! Stop it," I said, "come on, don't cry you can look in your own time. It takes time to reclaim your body again. You are so beautiful."

I looked down, smugly. I could see flatness, I was like, "Whoa! I've had a tummy tuck."

"Have you looked then?" she asked inquisitively.

"Yes, Candy Pops, I have looked several times and I love my breasts and my new flat stomach," I then went on to say, "yep they have done a fantastic job and I cannot stop looking."

I went on to say that the zip support bra I wore allowed me to have a sneak preview throughout the day.

I went on and on, "Candy Pops," I called. While I was rambling on, I noticed that she had not replied or spoken for about two minutes. Candy Pops was deep in thought as she fixed her stare to the empty visitors chair by her bedside. She was not going to get any sympathy from me.

"Yes Verna?" she replied, as she forced herself out of the trance.

"Well," I started hastily, "Have you thought about women?"

I paused as she looked at me confused.

I then went on to say, "Well, why has a man got to want you? Why has a man got to be the one to approve?"

She glared at me in amazement, her eyes widened almost as though two horns had suddenly grown on the top of my head.

Unfazed I went on, "So why is it that you feel that you must have a relationship with a man? Why a man? Have you considered a woman? You are an attractive lady with so much love to give. Have you thought about a nice young lady? I work with some beautiful ladies you know. Consider a partner or companion. All you need is someone reliable, to love and care for you. It's not all about men, Candy Pops, it's not just about men at all."

* * *

My thoughts go out to those who have lost their fight for life to this silent killer.

Special dedication to miracle workers, that is what all the staff in the NHS and caring professions are.

I love every member of the staff at St Margaret, Princess Alexander and Broomfield Hospital. You have made a difference in my life and in the lives of others. I told many of you at the time how much I loved you for the work and commitment you have shown. You work so tirelessly, making sick people a little more comfortable, you know who you are.

The dark night shift on Oxo cube ward

I could hear the laughter, the undertones and the general chitter chatter of the dozen nurses that gathered around the nurses' station for their handover as it came to the end of their shift. I could hear the updates, the medical progress and the relaying of the progress of the day. Once fully briefed they left for the day to be with their friends and families.

The night shift arrived and so did the dark.

"Hrm, I need to take your blood pressure," I looked up and could figure out a nurse who sounded forceful. Her mission was to complete her rounds as quickly as possible, she held the sheet so tightly in front of her face... it rose with her breath.

"Okay," my voice disturbed with exhaustion. I felt a cold shiver, there was no introduction or warm vibes. I lay helplessly vulnerable feeding on oxygen, drains and drips, I looked to the side of my right arm and there were blue, red, green and yellow wiring, it was then that I realised that I had to keep calm, very calm to avoid blowing myself up. I looked around and the nurse disappeared without a whisper of good night.

Within minutes I heard the footsteps. I looked up and I could see it was that nurse again. Nurse Booby One grabbed my left arm without warning, placed the blood pressure belt around my arm and reached across to attach a clasping device designed to test my blood pressure through my fingertips.

The clasp was so tight it was cutting off my blood supply.

"May I move it to my toe?" I asked.

This was yanked off my fingers and placed on my left big toe.

Without warning a hard pencil type device was at the entrance of my ear before being prodded to my left ear, there was no ringing or clicking just a firm press against my ear, a five second pause then she was off. What the fuck! I shook my head in disbelief, I felt like a cow at a cattle market.

"Which thigh do you want your jab in?"

Oh no, it's her again.

After negotiating my arm to even out the pain, "Nope. Thigh," she insisted refusing to bend any rules. Frustrated at the lack of consistency, she raised my right leg and chose this on my behalf.

This felt like I had received a whopping great bee sting with compliments. Was I to have this every night for the duration of my stay? I thought, every night, Gosh. Fear filled my heart. Would I be brave enough to endure this torture?

I was told to drink plenty of water, which I did, to flush out the baddies, frustrated at the overfilled colostomy bag this would give them extra work. What an inconvenience!

If I weren't so ill, I would have emptied my piss myself. But I am ill and need your assistance that's why I am here. I am so sorry that you are underpaid and overworked, but I am ill and so dependent on you.

Throughout the night, full of fear, I wondered, is this where the story ends? No way, no way, I affirmed.

I could hear Nurse Booby One and Nurse Booby Two fumbling around the night shift.

'Where is bed eleven's notes?' Booby One would shout to Booby Two. Oh my God, what a night. Throughout the night my hearing sharpened. This behaviour was in for the night, all night, I could hear, where is this, where is that. Both nurses gave the impression that they were missing items of instruments and were ill prepared for their shift.

Booby Two raised serious doubts when she struggled with her iPhone.

It was clear that her night vision was not as good as it used to be and she would often place the device to the window to obtain better lighting.

Oh my god, Oh my god...

Whenever the Boobies came to tend to me I literally struggled and found strength, turned the light on despite my pain to assist the best way I could. I did not care that it was 2.30am in the morning. I just wanted the job done as my confidence in the Boobies diminished.

Throughout this anxiety my blood pressure alarm went sky high to an unacceptable level.

This raised the alarms throughout the ward and fed through to the nurses' station. Red flashing lights, beep, beep, beep, the sound went on and on. What is happening? I panicked but I could not move.

Flat on my back.

I waited and waited and waited. Nobody was coming to rescue me.

I raised my shoulders as high as I could and dug my shoulder blades deep in the soft mattress, struggling I managed to hoist my head up to see what was going on. There was no one around; I wondered whether the nurses were going to ignore the alarm, perhaps turn it off centrally. Would I make it through the night?

I peered over to Stella over the other side of the ward. I could hear snores from the deepest of sleep, clearly unable to assist.

Dusky was oblivious, not a sound or movement from my right.

Oh my God, I thought in panic, what can I do? I quickly tried to remind myself that I must be in safe hands, after all I was in hospital surrounded by the care staff, the doctors and the lovely nurses. What could go wrong? But then doubt overcometh; the thought of being in safe hands was short lived, the reality took over...

What were they doing, sleeping? I hissed in anger to myself.

The alarm in the ward kept on flashing red and beeping loud; it was mental. How could anyone in their right mind ignore this alert from a high dependency ward. This went on for a good four mins. Unbelievable!

"Hello... Hello? Are you alright?" a meek voice came from the other side. My name is Jeanette, are you alright?"

"No, I am not, I don't know what is happening. I can't move and my blood pressure monitor has raised up..."

"Ok, don't worry, I have just pulled my alarm too. Hopefully someone will come soon. I can't move otherwise I would come over and help you," she said.

Oh my god, I thought, blind leading the blind. Both of us flat on our backs unable to help each other. What a scenario.

After a short time Booby Two appeared, as calm as a river stream. Four minutes seemed like four hours... BITCH, I uttered under my breath, I watched her angrily as she walked in slow motion.

She walked slowly over to Jeanette first, "Have you pulled the alarm?" she asked. "Why? Why have you pulled your alarm?"

I heard Jeanette's gentle voice say, "That lady over there needs you, her alarm went on, please help her..."

Nurse booby Two turned off her alarm and then walked over to me. There was no hurry, no urgency and no concerns displayed. It was as though she had headphones in, listening to opera...

My concerns were heighten alongside my flipping blood pressure.

She adjusted the alarm to reset it. I watched her every move in sheer amazement, I don't know why there was no urgency in her actions. I plucked up the courage to question her, well, what's the worst that can happen now, I thought. I egged myself on to be brave.

"Where were you?"

She didn't answer.

"Answer me," I pleaded, "Why did you take so long? Were you asleep? Some Intensive care unit," I looked at her, she looked at me oblivious to my anger. I said, "I could have had a stroke, you took your time, is this not a high dependency ward?" I asked sarcastically, "I needed you to help me?"

She tutted, "Don't be silly, you would not have had a stoke..."

I insisted and tried to justify my anger with her, "My father passed away through a stroke." How the hell would she know... she didn't care, she just wanted to get through the night shift.

Throughout the night I could hear the Boobies together, I daren't sleep, how could I?

Nurse Booby Two appeared to be unable to read the writing written by the last nurse, she was not discreet about this and everything was discussed within earshot. It alarmed me immensely.

How did she think she could write an accurate record if she could not read what was written before?

Did she think because I was ill that I had lost my hearing too? I felt insignificant, I no longer had a voice. I was just the patient in bed 11.

Nurse Booby One was too old for this new technology age, I wondered how she managed to get through her training. I grew more and more lacking in confidence, I wondered when she last had her eyes tested. I watched in disapproval as she struggled to read the screen on the iPad.

I grew more and more concerned. I would say, "Don't worry darling, just turn on the light." For me this was to assist the accuracy of the reading, I had to manage my destiny. I've been fighting for my life so far, the fight was not over yet, the night staff exhausted me.

Fuming, I waited intensely for the day staff to arrive and start their shift, I was poised, ready to pounce like a child missing their parents having been left with the babysitter.

I watched as night turned into day. The birds started to sing their morning song, the traffic outside sounded lounder and louder, there was an injection of life inserted into the ward. I could hear the voices of the day staff, as they peeped in the ward, I was so glad as the freshness filled the air.

How dare they leave me with the Bad Nurse Boobies of the night.

I felt justified in questioning their judgement for all of our sakes.

"Nurse Angel, Good morning, thank you for coming back to look after me. I am tired now and need to sleep I didn't get any sleep last night."

I went on to relay the events of the night as Nurse Angel stroked me to sleep.

I began, "The Bad Boobies came last night."

"What do you mean?" said Angel.

I relived my experience with the Boobies, tears ran down my face, as I relived the pain and the frustrations they caused me, as if I was not sick enough.

I struggled to catch my breath, I was exhausted. I pleaded, "Angel, please do not leave me with them tonight. I don't feel safe."

I think my pain and frustrations transferred into her soul. I did not need to say anymore. She knew.

I asked Nurse Vanisha about her family, she revealed that she was unable to bear a child. Her patients were her children. This showed in her approach and magical healing touch.

As she tucked me in securely, her bare arms were revealed I reached over unannounced, and fulfilled my compulsion and kissed her arm in gratitude.

"Angel I love you. Thanks for coming back to look after me."

"Angel?"

"Yes Verna?"

"I have started to write a book."

"Aww, that's good," she said sympathetically.

"Angel."

"Yes Verna?"

"Is there evidence of my illnesses? Is there evidence of what I have just gone through, has everything been documented?"

"Yes Verna it has."

"It's just that they won't believe me... Angel it's just that right now I feel that no one would believe what I have been through!!"

She listened intently to my troubles and concerns as she plumped up the pillows underneath my head and tucked me in securely underneath the layers of thin sheets.

She smiled as her beautiful red hair beamed in the sun's rays, "I love you and thanks for looking after me."

Angel's presence was felt as she pottered efficiently around the ward, nothing but care and compassion was oozing from her presence, reassured. It was then that I felt safe enough to catch up on some overdue sleep.

* * *

Dr Waring, Dr Julia and Dr Raja gathered together in my quarters. Dr Waring pulled the curtains shut for privacy and five minutes of entertainment from me, this eccentric patient, I had my audience.

I fumbled to switch off Drake's energy coarse lyrics from my iPhone but it was too late, I think it was too late, Dr Waring caught sight of my rebellious streak.

I managed to rip off the headphones attached to my head and pay attention. With a view of detaching myself from my secret passion.

"Well, Der der der der der..." They said in their speech

"What does that mean?" I asked in my efforts to participate and to be part of the conversation. You know, show an interest and learn some medical facts about my ordeal.

Despite breaking it down, I was none the wiser. I don't know why I was asking, I was none the wiser just more confused.

As I relayed lasts night's experience, no way I could let it go. A night with the Boobies, oh my God why were they allowed to allegedly look after me. I wanted an answer from Dr Waring as I questioned, he in turn mimicked by holding his fingers up to his ears and indicated Micky Mouse ears we all laughed it off. Dr Waring you were so real and so human, just the ideal medicine, the ideal tonic that I needed, you had me and your colleagues in absolute hysterics.

Thank you, may the light shine on you.

After a thorough inspection of their work and approval of the healing process, the curtains were pulled back and a serious stance was again undertaken, it was business as usual.

Nurse Jo and Nurse Diana

"Can you believe it?" Again I recalled my night with the Nurse Boobies experience, for those of you who know me, know that I am not one to let things go that easily.

Nurses Booby One and Booby Two, I hope this message has got back to you both in a positive way.

Change your attitude. I laid helpless, temporarily. When you move my water jug, please be mindful and place it back. I couldn't reach it after you left due to the pain and inabilities and I had to call you again and again, you made me feel as though I was a nuisance! I was not a nuisance, I was in need and dependent on you.

The Team

Dr Julie – Attractive mixed race of White/Chinese origin. She was well spoken and talented. She had dark straight shoulder length hair, not a kink or curl in sight, chiselled features and a warm nature.

Mr Griffiths – Charming, gifted and a proven expert in his field as top surgeon. He had blonde hair spiked up as though he had run his hands through his hair a thousand times throughout the day. Clean shaven with perfect red lips, he was gentle and displayed real passion for his work. He was that boy mechanic that pulled me apart and placed every piece of me back together again.

Dr Waring – Dark, handsome and tenacious. Boyish charm of excitement and naughtiness. He had dark spiky cropped hair, piercing blue eyes disguised behind his thick black framed glasses.

Dr Raja – Exactly like Raj Koothrappali from the *Big Bang Theory*; very charming, witty, unassuming and trustworthy, again well deserving of his title of fellowship.

Thanks for inspecting my broken body, and mending it… not sure that I wanted you to at the time. I now know that there was no other way, I had no choice as I reluctantly submitted myself to you. I allowed you to draw, plan and observe and together you planned my reconstruction.

When I told you that I wanted a sexy body, like Whoop whoop! 38, 34, 38, you listened and delivered to perfection… without prejudice.

You did not judge me, but worked with me. Through your gifted healing hands, your talent and determination prevailed. I Thank you all so very much.

I am so grateful that you have given me back my body, thanks for cutting out the badness and filling me with the good. I have taken this to move forward in my life and to be a better person.

All is mine to face.

The Pain

Artery or vein

At this time they tried to insert the cannula into my left arm and I am not exaggerating when I say that they tried every visible vein in my arm and each time they either missed the vein or the vein collapsed. My God by the end of it I was covered in 'Jook jooks'.

Every time they put the needle in, they would try to reassure me and would always say 'sharp scratch' just as they're doing it.

I would brace myself, cringe, stiffen, imagine the needle and then I told myself not to be silly. I did this hundreds of times over and over; it did not make it any easier for the next time.

Jook jooks, what thigh tonight? Every night for seven nights an injection to prevent DVT, plus two every daytime that stung like bee stings.

I hated every minute of this, but the choice was out of my hands.

Just going to take blood echoed, throughout my stay... blood, injections, take blood, blood, blood, blood.

What blood test?

What injection?

"For Pete's sake leave me alone," I pleaded as I counted all the bruises inflicted around my body.

A man in a blue uniform with a badge shuffled over to my bed. He disturbed my catheter again, as he stepped on it through incompetence. It twisted and the urine was not feeding through, until I felt an uncomfortable sensation of cystitis...

Who is this buffoon! I asked, he must be staff as he was in uniform and he had a name badge.

He said something... I couldn't understand what he was saying.

He then indicated that he was there to take blood. Oh for God's sake, I thought, so fed up with this constant violation. I watched him flit from arm to arm as he struggled to get blood from my left arm.

He went over to my right arm and took my blood from there, it was horrible as he fussed around to seek the best vein. After tapping for the vein to reveal itself he sought the assistance from tying a strap to my arm.

I wanted to cry and scream all at the same time, but I don't think I would get away with it. I am not a baby anymore.

I wanted to hold his hand while he inserted the needle, I was scared. I tried to think of a scratch but this thought was overtaken by the sheer truth... no!

After a short while the process was completed until another three hours.

The man in blue packed up from there and off he went. I later learned that he should not have disturbed that side of my right arm.

How was I to know... Who was he?... I found myself mentally preparing for an ID procedure should this be necessary to locate the suspect later on.

It was Mr Bella, an oversees doctor. Italian speak English... when I saw him I pretended I was asleep, but there was no escape, there was no warning, he didn't mention any sharp scratch, he was brutal. He would just pull my arm and abstract blood. I was frightened, frustrated and helpless and felt very vulnerable and violated.

As I relayed his description in case it was needed for evidence later on, I was growing very tired and weary. I needed to switch off and rest.

An hour later a lady stood in the middle of the room. She had the haematology uniform that I recognised. White with red piping.

"Hello!" I could see that she was checking my bed number above my head, "I've come to take your blood," she exclaimed.

"Pardon!" As I took deep breaths to pace my anxious anxieties, my blood pressure was rising fast.

She repeated "I have come to take blood."

I looked around to see if there were any cameras lurking around... *Trigger happy TV* came to mind... Would they do such a prank in a hospital full of seriously ill people?

"Nah man! Is this some sort of sick joke? Right!" I could feel my worst behaviour seeping out. "Who was that an hour ago in blue?" My voice took an authoritative tone, I shouted at the top of my voice? "Who was it?" I turned to the other sick patients in the ward, "Did you see who that was?"

My voice become louder as I held the ward to ransom, I went into panic mode.

My mind began to over load. Was he an imposter? Is there a sick maniac on the loose taking blood or worse, injecting vulnerable patients!

After the alarm was raised and I turned the clear air blue with obscenities, the male in blue was located by the nurses and certified as a genuine doctor. He was from Italy working as a locum GP.

English was not his first language, I was assured that this was work in progress.

Thank you for travelling from your homeland to assist and thank you for your efforts to help us to maintain an efficient NHS service, the reality of this crisis is finally sinking in.

I felt like absolute crap, I was tired and mega depressed about having to stay overnight in this hellhole away from my family and friends. A new lump of shit to deal with, typical, just what my nerves needed! Little did I know that this was the least of my worries and it was actually the neighbour in the next bed alongside me that would make me want to hang myself from my IV pole.

I felt as though I was fighting a battle without a shield.

I was in the forefront, ill-equipped.

Everything hurt, the light in my eyes, the pain in my head, the stench of blood in my nostrils, my hands were sticky with it.

"Verna," The voice comes dim through the fog of pain, I tried to shake my head, my lips won't form the word.

"Verna, you are safe in the hospital, we are giving you your medication."

Jamesha

"Hello. My name is Jamesha," I looked up and saw the petite female who introduced herself to me.

"Hello, Jamesha, how are you darling?"

"I am fine, I've come to take your temperature and change your dressings," she announced in broken English as she lovingly moved her head from side to side.

"Thank you darling, thank you so much for looking after me."

"This is why I am here, I've come to look after you." She did too, all the way from India.

"I came from India with my husband, we both decided that we wanted to come here to work for the NHS. He works here too in this hospital as a porter. We have been in this country for three months now. As she reminisced about her past life in India her eyes were fixed as though she was back home.

Intrigued, "How did you become a trainee nurse in this country?"

She then diverted her attention back to me.

"At home I was a care worker, I am training to be a nurse, so I go to university and three days a week I..."

"Oh like a day release?"

"Yes, Yes," she confirmed, "like day release, I like my job and I am learning everyday. I studied in Cambridge and have now I moved here for a while, I have to go to different hospitals for experience."

Her English was amazing, her touch was gently to perfection. I didn't care where she came from, she was warm and caring and I, we needed her.

I was totally helpless and dependent.

She was to assist me in taking my first independent shower. Oh my god, this was such a big task. Raw and wounded after being brutally mutilated, I slowly walked to the shower room aided by Jamesha, shackled with four drains still inserted in my body. I was led carefully to the washroom.

For a short while I was like a prisoner, acquitted but still held on remand from this awful disease. I stripped off to my flesh and bandages to have my first shower. Jamesha removed my dressings carefully.

I sat on this specially adapted chair and gripped the rail as tight as I could, I feared fear. If I fell over, I would not be strong enough to get back up. I was now disabled. It dawned on me that I had temporarily lost my independence and I could not complete even this simplest of tasks.

The shower splashed and then I felt the warm sensation of the water against my skin, the cleansing of the water and the sweet smell of the soap, I felt like a helpless child as Jamesha carefully tested the temperature.

I felt that I was being washed for the first time by my mummy.

"Jamesha, Jamesha," I quickly reverted to my sternest of voices, "Please don't wash my hair, do you hear me! Do not wet my hair as they are hair extensions and I cannot get them wet, it will take hours to dry and we have not got the facilities here."

She looked at me wide-eyed, she nodded in understanding as she took my requests through her eyes almost like a radar.

Jamesha saw the desperation in my face, whether or not she fully understood the full extent in my request, it must have been the part when my teeth became fangs, she knew there would be trouble if she disobeyed she tilted her head from side to side in understanding.

After about an hour and 15 minutes, I suddenly came over to this rush of unconsciousness I was overwhelmed by the steam. I remember feeling very weak and vulnerable as I drifted in and out of consciousness, desperately trying to control it.

"Jamesha!" I pleaded, "Help me, help me. I am slipping away". I was prepared to leave that bathroom wet, naked with soap suds still over my face and body. I must get out of here. I was losing control.

"It's ok," she said.

"Let me out now?"

"It's ok, ok," she said so calmly. "Just breathe in, out, in, out."

As I followed her breathing pattern, she placed the towels over my back and held them in place over my shoulders, she then held me tightly, I felt a great sense of reassurance, I caught her arm as she tried to hoist me up before kneeling in front of me to dry my body, I kissed her arm in appreciation.

"Thank you Jamesha, I love you very much and I am so grateful, I really am."

She moved her head from side to side and simply acknowledged my appreciation.

"Thanks ok, I am here to look after you."

This is the longest shower that I have ever had, it must have been around two whole hours.

To my Indian sisters who have left their families to travel from your homeland seeking work within the NHS England. Thank you.

Good News: It's Final

No chemo.

No radio.

Just carry on.

I won't pretend that the experience has not changed me, it has. It has definitely taught me a lot and opened my eyes to things I wouldn't have necessarily noticed or given a second thought to before.

It has taught me a hell of a lot about compassion, after spending lots of time in hospital. Seeing lots of other people suffering, has given me much more than I ever had.

The feelings I had for these people were strong and although I already knew cancer affected millions of people's lives, seeing it first hand on these people around me and their families hit home and I knew the true meaning of compassion.

Thank you, thank You, thank you. My life was in your hands. In great appreciation, the only way I knew how, I grabbed Mr Patel's hands without implied permission or notice and kissed them as though they were priceless jewels.

I am lucky, make yourself lucky, be good to yourself and take actions to ensure longevity.

I did... You can.

Nurse Booby One and Booby Two

You inspired me to write this book.

You were both so awful, I need to tell all to those who may feel that they have to suffer in silence.

My job is to break up this silence and advocate for those unable to help themselves.

Thank God I have my independence back. I feel that I can now breath under water.

Now please do what you are supposed to do.

It's so hard when you have to rely on others to help you to do basic tasks, like pass the water jug to relieve your thirst.

I felt all the frustrations at once building up inside my stomach combined with an ever-rising blood pressure which was making my face hot and sweaty.

I couldn't reach to scratch my back.

I couldn't brush my hair with those night sweats.

You stepped on my catheter so many times, by accident?

I had to wait in pain before I could get your attention to correct this.

Unbeknown to you, when you moved my trolley to administer my drugs, you didn't put it back.

I struggled to reach for water after you had gone. I was hurting in my efforts so I had to call you back, I know you were busy and understaffed. But what could I do? I was helpless.

I could hear you throughout the night when you couldn't find the temperature monitor. I refused to sleep when you couldn't read your colleague's last recorded entry on my drains.

You said out loud that you couldn't read the writing on my drain. Oh no, no, no, what do you mean?

I jumped up like Lazareth, but was forced down again due to the heavy medication that overtook my strength. I refused to sleep because I was scared that this would allow you to take over completely.

I was so alert my hearing became sharp, I listened for every footstep and instrument. Once a cop, always a cop.

I had to pace myself and use my experience to highlight any shortcomings, I was not going to be a victim.

Nurse Boobies, this is only positive constructive feedback to help improve the service you deliver.

What a price I had to pay for this real life experience.

NHS: Please don't leave me, I need you!

"Dr Waring! Where are you going?" I woke up and caught the back of his blue tunic. It was him, his Etonian finely tuned accent, dark hair, glasses and his handsome face could not go amiss...

"I am going to the strike," he replied in a calm manner.

"But, but you are not a junior doctor, you are a middle doctor, it's only for junior doctors," I proclaimed, "so could you stay and look after me please, we need you in here?" I waited eagerly for his response, as I tried to barricade him with my presence still holding on to my two drains in my pillow case.

He looked at me, with that a look of pity and compassion.

"Yes Verna, I promise, I will look after you," and off he went... out of sight. What could I do in my vulnerable state?

Confused I watched him disappear into the melee, I presume he went outside to join his fellow workers and protestors, after all I was confined to my OXO Cube ward. I was weak and could not walk any further to convince him nor his colleagues to stay.

From Overseas

Thank you for travelling from overseas. I don't know how I would have coped with a shortage of qualified staff. There is a strike on, what bad timing to be ill.

Police for Nurses

I looked up, I saw the tea ladies dressed in green.

"Morning, would you like tea or coffee?"

"Coffee please and a slice of toast please."

Gosh I was starving, there is nothing worse than waiting to be fed.

Time to sit up and see my day nurses. I could smell the sweet aroma from Angel before I saw her.

"Verna," she said sympathetically, "Did you get plenty of sleep? What have you been doing last night, you look absolutely exhausted? Did you get a good night's sleep? You do know that you need plenty of rest, especially after what you have been through." She then went on to say, "The drains measurements have not moved and I am not happy."

I rubbed my bloodshot eyes and looked up upon hearing that familiar voice. She came closer to conduct her daily checks and pulled out her thermometer. I looked at her closer and could see the many lines that formed in her forehead, as she frowned in disappointment.

"What's wrong?" I asked.

"Your drains are still at 40."

"Fourty, what does that mean?" I asked.

"Der de der de der der der Blah blah Blah!" She explained... dazed and confused I was still none the wiser other than the fluids were not draining as well as they should have and my blood pressure was higher that it should have been.

"Angel?"

"Yes," she replied in her sweet voice

"I have a confession to make?"

She looked at me attentively as she drew close up to my bedside.

"Well," I began, "I know that you are going to be disappointed with me."

She came closer to my bedside and listened attentively, "There was a disturbance last night and there was a lot of shouting from the nurses station, I was intrigued so I struggled and got up and walked towards the window of Oxo cube ward, I opened the door and listened."

"Go on," she nodded.

"Well, I was spying through the door which was I left ajar... I busied myself as I carried my drains in my efforts to find out what was going on, but was really exhausted. I think I've overdone it and my stomach hurts."

I then began my story, "Last night there was a lot of screaming and shouting. There was an old girl from the ward next door, she must have been around 80 years of age. She was screaming, swearing and shouting out really loudly, it must have been around 1.40am.

"Go on," she encouraged.

"Well, from what I could gather, she wanted to go home, I could hear the nurses trying to persuade her to stay the night and settle down. I heard her using all the foulest of swear words, she really sounded full of anger and rage."

"Angel, you know that in her frustrations she must have forgotten that she was disturbing a ward full of very, very sick, gravely ill patients. Unbelievable is all I can say, absolutely Angel, you couldn't make it up.

"Listen here, ole girl, how could you. I would love to show you a video clip of your behaviour! You nearly made history as I contemplated your arrest for public order."

"My God, ole girl I would have had to reveal myself. I had my warrant card in my bag ready to act, do you know ole girl that it could have happened at anytime, even though I still had the drains attached to me."

"How would I have conducted this arrest? Would I have sufficient grounds I ask? How would I have detained her, how would I have written my arrest notes and obtained witness statements? Would I call the nearest nick to get assistance?"

I wondered if the body worn cameras have been rolled out yet... I questioned and questioned to absolute exhaustion, I felt light headed and I could no longer stand.

"I slowly gripped my slippers with my toes, once my feet was placed firmly inside, I slowly made my way back to my bed. I stooped over to my handbag and tucked my warrant card safely back into my bag, I slowly climbed into bed and pulled the covers over my head." I looked at Angel, somewhat smugly, so there you have it... I waited in anticipation for Angel's reaction.

"Verna."

Knowing Angel was going to tell me off, I interrupted her quickly to disrupt this.

"Angel who were the nurses in red? Were they the nurse police? I saw quite a few of these Nurses running backward and forward in the ward."

Angel smiled sweetly and knowingly, "They are admission nurses, but they probably came last night to assist in calming the disturbance."

"Angel, does this type of thing happen often?"

Non-committal, she shrugged her shoulders. Angel replied, "not really," in her efforts to reassure me.

"Angel."

"Yes, Verna?"

"What happens in situations like this, do you call the Police?"

"No," she replied. "No, not at all, we simply speak calmly and diffuse situations down, don't we?" she asked.

I nodded in acknowledgment, understanding the use of her language, "Of course we do."

For a short while I lost my identity.

The little red book

Still in disbelief.

I sat up in bed admiring the silence and the calm.

For the first time in ages I peered down and watched my chest rise and fall with my breath.

I touched my wrist with my finger tips and felt that calm beat of my heart.

I took in a deep breath of contentment and as I decided to spend the early part of the morning reading, I reached over to my bedside cabinet.

I realised that my little red book was missing... I couldn't see it anywhere, I searched, got up and searched the bed, I then checked my suitcase, the cabinet again, under the bed, I grabbed the bed and unruffled it in a desperate attempt to find my red book.

"Where is my book?" I said out loud. I could feel my eyebrows lowering to reach my eyelids.

"Who has taken my book?" Again, in my delirious desperate state I asked again who has taken my book.

"Oh for fucks sake," I ranted.

I did not realise that I was speaking loudly at this point, it did not feel real. It did not feel as if the words were coming out of my mouth. Did I lose my manners? I am not normally this rude and outspoken in a respectful place.

Seething I hissed, "You better find it," I promised to any random person present who was concerned enough to listen and get involved.

I felt that I was in a girls' dormitory at school.

Concerned, the nurses searched the whole ward rushed over to me and in an effort searched all the bins and the linen baskets.

Nurse Diana again searched the bed and found my precious book.

"There you are," she said in her soft firm perfectly formed elocutionary tone. "It's ok."

The relief and delight was felt by everyone as I expressed my deepest gratitude to all involved in this Stop 'n Search exercise.

Sister Jo came along three hours later, "Where is that damn book." The serious tone in her voice told me that I was being told off. She went on to say, "We had searched everywhere and turned all the linen out. Please leave it there on top of your table so we can see it."

I looked down in shame at her beautifully polished court lace up shoes, her neatly pressed tunic, her belt and then our faces met. As both our eyes met our smiles could not be contained any longer.

Our belly laughs developed fully and could no longer be contained or masked as we both burst out in full laughter together like an explosion of fireworks. How pathetic on the scale of things...

Goodbye, it's time to leave

Dusky
"Verna."

"Yes, Dusky?"

"I have been allowed to go tomorrow."

"Aww Dusky, gonna miss you."

"Come on my bed for your leaving party." We shared a cup of water and went through our phones sharing photos of our individual life achievements.

Your family that you spoke of so proudly came to collect you to take you home. We didn't kiss, you left as quickly as you came. Softly!

Stella
"Bye!"

"Thanks for your contact number."

"Look after yourself."

She disappeared as fast as she came, "No emotions please, I don't want to cry." She said quickly.

"Me too," I whispered.

Jeanette

You gentle lady, I'll never forget your kindness. It was the blind leading the blind.

You wrote your contact number in my book. Thank you, it's in a safe place. We kissed and said goodbye. Did you notice the radio playing *Walk On By* as you left the room?

Candy Pops

"It was me and you, kid." The dynamics were changing vastly.

We learned how to dance as Nurse Diana and Nurse Jagger played the radio as they remade the now vacant beds. Who were we getting now, we wondered?

I've come down from my high now.

"Candy Pops," I asked concerned, "can you feel it, the dynamics have changed." I felt that it was now time to reflect.

Motown, Diana Ross, our favourite came on. *Chain Reaction.*

The nurses opened the show as they displayed their dancing skills. They were very successful in their attempts at keeping our spirits up. This in itself was enough reason to dance our troubles away.

I felt a sense of honour and humbleness. I did not manage to dodge the bullet of cancer, but fell softly after the blow.

Candy Pops then invited me to dance with her as she hung onto her drains, I grabbed mine as we both stared at each other with sheer determination. Both determined to get back to normal. We carefully moved slowly side to side, careful not to disturb our stitches. Both of us gliding like Tin Men, the strength of the medication proved to be pain proof. We reminisced and psyched ourselves up for our imminent release and departure, freeing us to go our separate pathways.

Marvin Gaye – *Let's Get It On.*

Cyndi Lauper – *Girls Just Want To Have Fun.*

Sister Sledge – *Frankie.*

Frank Sinatra – *I Did It My Way* and *Fly Me To The Moon.*

Gertrude
You now have Stella's Bed.

Simply Bye...

Laura – Anaesthetist

"Hello Laura, fancy seeing you here."

"Hello, Verna."

"I am going home now," I declared, I felt my ordeal was now coming to an end.

"Verna, it's so unusual to see patients after their operation and hospital stay."

I felt special. How ironic, I thought.

"I'm leaving now," I said impatiently, as I felt the urge to get back to normality. "You were there at the beginning when I lost seven hours of my life. I remember grasping you with my right hand before experiencing the unknown."

"I am pleased for you," she replied modestly.

"Laura, this is the end, thank you for looking after me. Can I take your picture? I have decided to write a book; you and your colleagues have inspired me."

"Of course you can, of course," as she posed deservingly.

"Thank you, Laura. You helped to ease my pain, you stayed with me at a time of darkness, I was alone, bare and naked, you were there to help me through to the other side."

Mr Patel meets Aeki

Thank you, Mr Patel, I am free. Thank you for removing the shackles and setting me free and I am now allowed to continue my life again constructively.

The mastectomy and reconstruction has now taken place, I certainly wear the scars to show it.

Reunited with my Gals

Two weeks later we met up for our first physiotherapy session.

This was lovely as it was the first time we had met up since our operation. I glanced at Candy Pops first as I looked inside the waiting area over the other side of the room.

I walked in slowly taking time not to disturb any stitches in my stomach, as I got nearer there was Dusty, Jeanette and finally Stella. We all stood up and hugged and kissed each other like long lost friends. I wanted to announce to the waiting room of onlookers, we are sisters that have come through a journey together.

As we all sat in the physiotherapy room together, Louis the physiotherapist recalled all our names one by one, again united in this classroom environment.

As I looked around the room we all looked well. What a journey we had all been on as we mimicked Louis and raised our hands in their air to prove that we had done our exercises.

I thought that was it, as we all practiced our five point exercises. I thought we all did the distance.

I thought we were all in the clear. We didn't realise that there were more hurdles to jump. We all thought that was it.

After waiting anxiously for an hour in the surgery for my results, Nurse Alinson called me in.

"Hello, Mr Patel, I am here to hear the news, the results Mr Patel. What is it now, is it good news? Please, please finalise this pain and torture once and for all."

"Calm down, Verna otherwise you will not hear what I am about to say."

I felt my stomach open out ready to drop to the floor. I didn't think that I could physically and mentally cope anymore. Again Dave was to my right, but I daren't look at him. I didn't want to let him down anymore, never mind me, I don't think he could cope with anymore either... This moment seemed to last for a long time.

"I am pleased to tell you that the results are back. The cancer that you had was hormonal and we have treated this... I am now so pleased to tell you that you are all clear. The results are back and that's it. I do not have to see you for another year."

I was so happy the weight was lifted off my shoulders. Reduced to tears, I got up from my seat, reached over and kissed Mr Patel's arm. That was the only part I could reach. Unannounced as I grabbed his arm I said, "God Bless your hands" and raised my left hand and created a fist pump in the air as I reached over and kissed Dave and then Nurse Alura.

That's it, my time was up. I left the room motionless, ignoring the eyes of other patients waiting for a reaction or any indication of the news that I had received.

Chosen

Dusky, Jeanette, Candy Pops, Stella and Gertrude.

You all came into my life unexpectedly at a time of uncertainty, pain and loneliness.

We were strangers and came together through illness, we bonded and shared our stories and experiences, almost as though the universe had just randomly thrown us together. From different backgrounds the only common feature was that we all had cancer.

As we broke the silence and that thin layer of ice, Dusky revealed that she works at Homemaker Ltd. You look so young for your age, a doting yummy mum and nan.

Jeanette, a shop assistant in a local bakery certainly reflects all the sugar 'n spice and everything nice.

Candy Pops, a school assistant, I could tell by your caring nature, placing everyone before yourself. You brighten the room with your presence and sexy lingerie

Gertrude, you selfish soul, are you ready to come out and make friends yet?

Goodnight Nurse Booby One, Goodnight Nurse Booby Two. What a nightmare you both were. Thank God you are out of my life for good.

Good Morning, Angel. Thank you for coming to look after me. Your scent of sweetness, the aroma was smelt before I saw your pretty face. You were the calm over trouble waters.

Ms Dusky Dawn

Heterosexual.

Dob 02/06/1980.

Lives in Waltham Abbey.

Single mum.

One daughter, one son.

Works at Homemakers Ltd.

New grandmother of four months old baby, first grandchild Calum.

Dusky was so easy to get on with, nothing was too much trouble. She looked younger than her years and when we got talking she was so funny she didn't even know it. She had me in hysterics and possessed a positive genuine nature.

I had only known her for five days.

Dusky was straight down the line and very honest what you saw was what you got.

Dusky was finally finding peace, inner peace in life after a long dysfunctional relationship with her ex partner; violence and unreliability fuelled with excessive alcohol and empty dreams.

She was frank and open as she recalled her life but still contented with her lot.

"I was here last year, I had a hysterectomy, there can't be much of me left now, oh well."

Now that's what I call genuine dry humour. I placed my hands over my mouth to contain the smile that developed into inappropriate laughter. The noise of hysterics could not be contained or drowned out, despite placing my hands tightly over my lips. I gave up and laughed hysterically at her blasé attitude, unable to control myself or my laughter.

I truly admire your sheer honesty and unpretentious attitude, Dusky, but hey, you're alive and living.

Thank you Dusky. When we sat in the filled room it was fate that we were put together to fulfil our journey.

Ms Candy Pops

Heterosexual.

Dob 26/02/1969.

Lives in Harlow.

Single mum.

Two grownup boys.

Works are a care assistant.

New grandmother of four months to baby Poppet.

Candy Pops has a larger than life personality and beams a ray of sunshine when she walks into the room.

I had known her for six days.

Candy pops is the salt of the earth and not shy to express how she feels, which is often coupled with F's and B's.

Despite her ordeal, she came with a full suitcase of a selection of nightwear including a silky sexy dressing gown.

"Oi," I shouted over to her, "where do you think you are going?" she swayed from side to side as she modelled this sexy attire together with her guest slippers and perfect makeup.

"Well," she replied, "you never know who you can find in here. There may be some fit doctors around!" It was then that it was confirmed that I had met my match. We spent the whole six days filled with laughter, trust and honesty.

Thank you, Candy Pops, I nearly forgot why I was in hospital after meeting you. You helped to ease the pain.

It is with great regret that I have to inform you that Candy Pops passed away on the night of 18th April 2017. She leaves behind sons Mitchell and Ryan and granddaughter Amelia.

Ms Jeanette Cream

Heterosexual.

Dob 01/10/1970.

Lives in Ockenden Essex.

Unknown.

Two grown up girls.

Works in the bakery department of a well known supermarket.

Jeanette possessed a quiet, gentle and calming personality.

I had known her for six days.

Jeanette was shy, polite and would not willingly participate in our coarse conversations, but would smile to confirm that it was ok. She was certainly no shrinking violet and would sporadically reveal her playful side discreetly.

Jeanette, thank you for your selfless attitude when the devils came on the night shift.

We both lay helpless, flat on our backs, but you still tried your best to assist and raised your alarm. I was in distress and needed someone, your soothing voice comforted me.

Thank you, Jeanette, towards the end you opened up and your personality beamed. There were so many things to say, but little time left to say it all.

Ms Stella Blonde

Heterosexual.

Dob 25/07/1965.

Lives in Woodford.

Divorced.

One grown up daughter.

Works as a PA for an Estate Agent.

Stella is from a large, close knit family of love, care and pampering.

I had known her for four days.

Stella appeared independent and this illness was clearly inconvenient, she needed to get back to work.

Stella recovered the slowest of the four of us, but when she came round you could see her true glamour and perfect figure.

It was clear that she enjoyed the finer things in life, such as good wine and travel; Portugal being one of her favourite places.

Stella, I am glad that somehow I gained enough trust from you, you have a 'no nonsense, don't suffer fools lightly' stature.

Thank you, Stella. I was always aware of your intriguing stares, watching you all the time and seeing the improvements you have made. You are remarkable.

Ms Gertrude Fonteleroy

Dob 05/09/1958.

Lives in La La Grange Palace.

Married Cuthbert Fonteleroy 20 years.

Two young boys.

Gertrude, you didn't get to know me and didn't allow me to call you Trudy! I ask, did you too have breast cancer? Probably you had a far more superior disease other than cancer? Is that why you kept your distance and drew your curtains closed?

Your actions were so selfish.

Did you know that we sisters have to fight together against cancer... It is indiscriminate, despite our cultures and background. All the riches in the world cannot prevent it when it raises its ugly head.

Gertrude, we had so much fun and laughter before you came into the ward like a dark cloud. You changed the dynamics of this happy ward filled with laughter, bonding and friendship. When you decided that you were ready to engage with us, unfortunately, it was too late, we had already moved on and secured our sisterhood.

Good luck Gertrude, I hope you learnt your lesson. Change your ways and your attitude, you missed out on so much...

Mr Rocky Star

Rocky you were so near and yet so far away.

You have been through so much with your wife, why didn't I know?

In my deepest hour, I become introverted and asked why are we so selfish in society nowadays that we choose ignore our brothers and sisters in need.

Your wife had undergone sixty-seven operations and six hospital visits. This is just part of your journey.

You have two young beautiful girls. It is our responsibility to ensure that you are managing and have someone to talk to.

Religious Sisters

Aadila tapped me quietly on the shoulder.

"Verna," she said, "I have read your book, it is really good and informative, did that really happen?"

"Thanks, Aadila. Yes it did," I immediately felt a warm a sense of pride and approval.

Confidently I went on to say, "Now, sis, tell me have you and your sisters had a ma..."

Without waiting for me to finish my question, Aadila immediately asked, "Was the radiologist male or female?"

I looked at her puzzled as I thought about her question. A male or female, why the hell would this matter, I thought. It then dawned on me that my best friend was a Muslim woman, something that I was totally oblivious to. I looked at her again in more detail; she was wearing her Hijab around her head and she dressed in dark clothing covering her arms and legs. I forgot she was a Muslim girl; of course her modesty was an integral part of her faith and religious practices. I was blind to this and only saw her as Aadila.

"Verna," she said in a stern, almost questioning voice as she maintained eye contact with me, "did you know that even today physical contact (e.g., hand-shaking) and eye contact with men may be unacceptable to some Muslim women, so I suppose that assigning same-sex caregivers could alleviate some of the stress of maintaining modesty in the healthcare setting and remove the possibility that the patient may refuse treatment from a male caregiver."

"Hmmm," I replied in agreement, "I never thought of it like that."

"I know that when my sister had certain examinations over her clothing or a hospital gown and in the presence of another female they were ok about this, she just looked at us as if we had grown two heads."

"Oh really, yes," I agreed as I listened intently.

Aadila went on to say, "If clothing must be removed for an examination, caregivers should expect some reluctance and ensure that the patient is given as much time as she needs to undress and feel comfortable before the examination begins.

Muslim women often do not seek out screening for cancers that require invasive procedures. Cancer is often undiagnosed or poorly controlled until serious complications arise. Paradoxically, the use of high-tech interventions for prolonging life is pushed beyond reasonable limits.

Did you know that I know one muslim woman ignored the cancer growing in her breast because she didn't want to risk a referral to a male doctor.

Another was divorced by her husband on the mere suspicion she had the disease, while a third was dragged away from a mammogram machine because the technicians were men."

I listened in disbelief and shook my head in pity. I needn't say anything, I didn't have to. The discussion of cancer within the Asian Muslim and other forgotten communities is very limited.

My Cypriot Friends

As I laid upstairs reminiscing, I heard Alex call from downstairs. "Mum, can my friends come to see you?"

"Yes of course, darling," I shouted down, I deepened my voice to reassure him that my strength was coming back.

I sorted the pillow from behind my head and made sure that I was decent to receive my guests.

"Yioddy, how are you darling? I felt real gratitude."

This little boy that use to play with mine is now a man.

"Hi, Verna. How you doing?" He asked, his voice was deep and broken.

"Yes, good, Yiod. I am getting there."

He then raised a bunch of beautiful, beautiful colourful flowers.

"Thanks, Yiod, my first flowers, they are so beautiful."

"That's, OK." He then went into a sheepish shy stance.

"I didn't know what card to get you, so I got you this one."

OK, two glasses filled with champagne.

"Verna, when you are better we can go to King William and take some shots yeah?"

"Oh yes, of course Yiod, of course, Thank you."

He then joined the rest of the boys downstairs.

I threw my dressing gown on and decided to join the boys.

"Carl, you OK, are you, my entertainer?" I asked. I was a bit confused. It was the anesthetic. Carl had been recuperating from a football injury. He continually placed his red stress ball on his nose, he did this sparingly, no one else seem to mind or comment.

"Am I going mad?" I asked myself.

He looked like a clown, I laughed hysterically. "Carl?" I said in a stern voice.

"Yes, Verna?"

"Are you a clown? Have you come to entertain me?"

He smiled sweetly without saying a word and oblivious to my question he continued to play with his red nose, placing it on and off his nose with the occasional squeeze for tension.

For God's sake, all I needed now was Brough to come as Father Christmas.

Booth was another friend off sick due to a broken foot injury. Home from home, I felt a sense of pride that my son knew that he needed to be close to his mother, so he brought his best man, Dem, who wasn't mobile due to one injury or another to our house to chill. You're the Greatest / Champion!

Good food, drink and good vibes were flowing and plentiful.

Boys thank you for being a good friend to your mate. My son.

You have supported him at this time when his mother was ill with this often stigmatised disease.

I have watched you all grow and prosper together.

Yiod, I am so grateful to be alive to receive my first bouquet of flowers from you in person. My son, you have been spared from placing these by my graveside.

Thank you son.

Όπως ήμουν πάνω στο δωμάτιο μου ξαπλωμένη, αναπολώντας, άκουσα τον Άλεξ να φωνάζει απο το ισόγειο. < Μαμά, μπορούν οι φίλοι μου να έρθουν να σε δούν;>

<Βεβαίως αγάπη μου> του φώναξα και έκανα την φωνή μου να ακουστεί δυνατά για να τον βεβαιώσω ότι η δύναμη μου ερχόταν πίσω.

Έφτιαξα το μαξηλάρι μου πίσω από το κεφάλι μου και έκανα σίγουρα ότι ήμουν αξιοπρεπής για να δεχτώ τους επισκέπτες μου

<Γιώτη πως είσαι αγάπη μου;> Ενιωσα πραγματικά τόση ευγνωμοσύνη!

Αυτό το μικρό αγορι που συνήθιζε να παίζει με το δικό μου αγόρι είναι τώρα ένας άντρας.

<Βέρνα γειάσου. Πώς είσαι;>Ρώτησε με βαθειά και σπασμένη φωνή.

<Ναι καλά είμαι Γιώτη. Προχωρώ..>

Αμέσως μετάμου έδοσε ένα όμορφο πολύ όμορφο μπουκέτο από λουλούδια.

<Ευχαριστώ Γιώτη, τα πρώτα μου λουλούδια, είναι τόσο όμορφα>

<Κανένα πρόβλημα > Στάθηκε κάπως αμήχανα ντροπαλά.

<Δεν ήξερα τι κάρτα να σας πάρω και γι αυτό πήρα αυτή..Δύο ποτήρια με σαμπάνια ... Βέρνα όταν θα είσαι καλύτερα θα πάμε στο King William και εκεί θα πιουμε ένα δύο ε;;>

<Ο!!Ναι, βεβαίως Γιώτ, βεβαίως, Σε ευχαριστώ>

Μετά πήγε κάτω με τα άλλα αγόρια. Φόρεσα την ρόμπα μου και αποφάσισα να πάω κάτω στα αγόρια.

< Carl είσαι καλά; Είσαι ο καλλιτέχνης μου;> ρώτησα με απορία. Ο Carl ανάρρωνε από μια βλάβη που είχε στο ποδόσφαιρο. Έβαζε την κόκκινη μπάλα που είχε για στρες πάνω στη μύτη του και το έκανε με φειδώ και κανείς δεν φαινόταν να νιάζεται να να λέει κάτι.

<Έχω τρελλαθεί > ρώτησα.. Φαινόταν σαν κλόουν, γέλασα υστερικά. < Carl> είπα με αυστηρή φωνή

<Ναι Βέρνα>

<Είσαι κλόουν; Ήρθες να με διασκεδάσεις;

Χαμογέλασε γλυκά χωρίς να πει λέξη και αγνοώντας την ερώτηση μου συνέχισε να παίζει με την κόκκινη μπάλα, τοποθετώντας την στη μύτη του πιέζοντας την συχνά.

<Προς Θεού το μόνο που χρειάζομαι τώρα είναι ο Brough να έρθει σαν Αγιος Βασίλης >

Ο Booth ήταν ένας άλλος άρρωστος φίλος του Αλεξ, με σπασμένο πόδι. Ένιωσα περήφανη που ο γιος μου ένιωθε ότι έπερεπε να ήταν δίπλα στη μαμά του, ώστε έφερε τον πρωτο κουμπάρο του Dem λόγω του τραυματισμού του στο σπίτι μας να ξεκουραστεί. Εισαι ο καλύτερος.

Καλό φαγητό, ποτό όλα ήταν γύρω μας.

Αγόρια σας ευχαριστώ που είστε καλοί φίλοι στο φίλο σας. Τον γιο μου. Του σταθήκατε σε αυτή τη δύσκολη στιγμή όταν η μαμά του ήταν άρρωστη με αυτή την ασθένεια που πολλές φορές στιγματίζει. Σας είδα όλους να μεγαλώνετε και να προοδεύετε μαζί.

Γιώτ είμαι τόσο ευγνώμων που είμαι ζωντανή να πάρω τα πρώτα μου λουλούδια από εσένα προσωπικά. Αγόρι μου τουλάχιστον δεν χρειάστηκε να τα φέρεις στο τάφο μου.

Σε ευχαριστώ αγόρι μου.

Robbery of the Grieving Process

Hey, I'm sorry for robbing you of the grieving process, grief mongering and for dodging the pity that you were preparing to show.

Auntie Bambi, Uncle Redding, Cousins Pom Pom, Niece Tinker Bell, Philip and Geeta,

Arthur and my so called best friends Luka, Jason, Ariana and Agatha.

I hadn't actually heard from you for over a year, I suppose you have been getting on with your lives.

I had, until cancer disrupted my life, but hey... It would have been another year before I saw you again. It would have come and gone and been another so called drama in my life.

It took just under three months from start to finish, precisely 5th February 2016, when I was diagnosed with breast cancer and the gruelling months of treatment.

I am telling you at this late stage because I am pleased to tell you it's over and dealt with. It's gone.

I could see and hear the intrigue, the sense of missing out on details of the procedures, treatments and the living pity process.

I got the many messages asking me if everything was OK and whether I had the results back yet from scans etc. I have written this book to save any awkward questions.

I am so sorry that I did not tell you sooner. There was no need, I had to go it alone. There was no reason for me to be scared. I had my real friends and family around. I am privileged, I can now see colours again.

Moving on now, I realise how lucky I am. I'll shut up now, I know I have so much to be grateful for.

The End

It was a Sunday morning, I woke from a really deep sleep. It must have been around 3.20am

I felt light and burden free, sharp and ready to go. I looked down to the side of my right breast as I had done since my operation, I couldn't see Aeki.

Aeki was not there, I could feel palpitations coming on as I started to get panicky. I started conducting a thorough room search in my desperation to find Aeki, my comforter, my crutch. This was not funny not knowing where he is.

Aeki, Aeki, where are you? I grabbed my husband and shrugged his T-shirt. My efforts to wake him succeeded, he woke up astonished and he said calmly, "What's the matter baby?"

"I've lost Aeki, I've lost Aeki," I repeated this around eight times. I picked up the bedding, looked under the pillows, lifted the duvet and eventually I had to ask Dave to get up out of the bed so that a satisfactorily bedroom search could be conducted.

"Sorry Dave, you are going to have to get up out of the bed now," He looked at me intensely, perhaps he thought that I had lost my mind and was having a breakdown.

"Oh my God, where is Aeki? He is missing, Aeki is missing." I could hear my voice getting more stern as it changed to an official tone. I'm not flipping joking now!

Where the hell is this flipping damn frog! This bedroom search for the missing frog became a military operation.

An official search was being conducted in my bedroom in Chigwell can you believe it! A search for a missing frog.

I felt desperate again in my best efforts to conduct this effective and thorough search. I stripped the bed, unfolded every bed dressing layer by layer. Where the hell is this blasted frog...? It became clear that this was going to a negative search. He was clearly not there. No evidence, not a trace of Aeki at all.

My frog had leaped out of my life and turned into a Handsome Prince.

Hello my Prince David. Thank you for being by my side.

What is the name of your Prince or Princess?

Pull back your curtains and open out to the world, your sisters need you.

Check You Out

Be Good to yourself, avoid the energy drainers and the sappers.

Cancer patients are not all oppressed. We are just battle fighters; the ones that get knocked in life and move on.

Help yourself to be happy and surround yourself with those who are positive and make you happy.

Ask yourself, how am I feeling today? As you embark on this life changing journey!

Indulge yourself the night before surgery with treatments, this could be to your favourite bar of chocolate, a nice meal at your favourite restaurant or a cosy fun filled night in with friends and family.

Get that manicure/pedicure, consider a cheeky bikini wax session. Girlfriends you want to look your best at all times even when you are unaware that your Crown Jewels are being revealed!

Wet wipes are so handy; keep your pride, sisters.

Visit the dentist and look after your teeth.

Get your hair cut to a manageable length/weave up, fix up.

Make sure you pack a silk scarf for your hair to avoid excess night sweat and tangles

And take a good hair brush.

Pack a couple of hair bands.

Pack ear plugs. Some of your ward friends may snore. Right, Candy Pops Foghorn!

Wear your makeup if you want to, your silent armour.

Pack makeup and casual clothes to leave with.

Keep an appointment diary for all follow up appointments and visitors.

Let friends and relatives be just that.

Regain control of your life, do all the things that you got up to on your bucket list.

Be proud of yourself and have a positive outlook, rely on yourself.

Keep in contact with your friends; out with the old, in with the new.

Remember, same path, different shoes.

Enjoy your life to its maximum. We all know that this is not a rehearsal.

Lightning Source UK Ltd.
Milton Keynes UK
UKOW05f1914190617
303701UK00001B/70/P